Born This Way

Questions and Answers About Being Transgender

DeAnna Bennett

Dedication:

This book is dedicated to MJ (Michael/Marie) Burch. One of the bright shining lights that left this plane of existence way too soon. I will always love and remember him/her.

Table of Contents

Introduction

There is much confusion, mystery, and (I like to think) mysticism about what the world calls "Transgendered." My name is now DeAnna Bennett and part of my "herstory" is that I was born transgendered and then transitioned at age 44 after 40-plus years of living as a man. I did all of this to simply unify with my brain's Gender Identity. My story has similarities to hundreds of other transgendered people. I was born a man, now I'm a woman, and am finally living the life I felt I was meant to live. In my life as a man, I was married for 25 years to 2 different women, and I fathered 3 children. I am also a Grandparent to 11 grandchildren.

My story and ultimately my decision to transition, begins in October of 1991. At this point in my life (as a man), I was serving in the US Army as a Field Artillery Captain during the first Desert Storm in 1991. I had served in the Army since 1983 as a commissioned officer. My unit was decisively engaged during this conflict, and my unit eventually fired over 3,000 rounds in combat. I received a Bronze Star that was awarded for courageous action serving as a commander during this combat operation.

I had an experience (see chapter 1) while sitting in the desert in the Middle East waiting to go to war. Approximately, a year after getting home from the Middle East I was offered an opportunity to get out of the Army and I decided to take it. I knew that whatever "this thing" inside me was, it was not going to go away and was only getting stronger, I also knew in my heart of hearts the Army wasn't going to be very understanding.

After leaving the service in 1992 I moved my family to the Phoenix area, and became a real estate appraiser. I even, at one point, put my paperwork in to become a Methodist minister.

I began openly transitioning my gender in the spring of 1999 by starting counseling, which is required for anyone seriously considering gender reassignment surgery. Early in this process I was directed to a couple of support groups. One was called Alpha Zeta (a cross-dressing group), and the other was called Transgendered Harmony (kind of an open catch all group, but was primarily Male To Female transsexuals). I eventually left Alpha Zeta, but ended up staying with Transgendered Harmony.

Eventually, I ended up taking on the leadership of the group (Transgendered Harmony) and today share that responsibility with two other good friends. Since 1999, I have addressed a wide variety of groups, beginning with the ministers of my own church, which was not really the most fun I have ever had. I remember them telling me that they were starting to become afraid of me, and where I appeared to be headed. I offered to have an "all church" meeting and I would explain it. They did not think that was an option. I went on to speak at colleges, at first with other members of the group, later on my own, addressing all aspects of being transgendered.

I've also taught a countless number of classes over the years while leading the group and still find it interesting that while information is more and more readily available, there is still much confusion, misinformation, and fear about this topic.

Being transgendered has been quite an eye-opening experience, and I have dealt with almost every aspect of this amazing human condition. During and after becoming a woman, I opened my home up to this community. Beyond my own personal transition experience, I have served in one capacity or another in Transgender Harmony, one of the longest running transgender support groups in the United States, and have spoken extensively on this topic at a growing number of colleges, churches, and other organizations.

One of the main components of my talks, at all the groups and classes over the years, has been an open question and answer period. I tell my audience, "This is your chance to ask any question you have ever wanted to ask of someone like me. I have never had a question I wouldn't answer, so go for it, there is no question I will not answer." The content of this book came about after years of answering interesting, real world questions from people just like you.

****DISCLAIMER: When speaking at colleges I like to thank the teachers for allowing me to tell the "story about me by me, rather than the story about me by NOT me." While I have had much experience with a large amount of the information please understand that everyone's journey is different. These are MY answers to difficult questions and it should be understood that there is never a totally correct answer to any of these questions. My journey has been as a MTF (Male to Female) transsexual. This is my experience. Much of what I will discuss has commonality with the FTM (Female to Male) but some will not.

This journey has been, for me, a very unique and powerful experience and continues to challenge me on so many new and different levels.

CHAPTER One: What's first? (the chicken or the egg)

1. The Big Question: Why did I personally make the decision to change my gender?

My story really begins sometime in late October/early November 1990 at a pretty dark moment in my life. The setting was in the Western Desert of Saudi Arabia in an area of the map labeled as "The Great Unknown." At the time I was known as Captain Dean Bennett and was an Artillery Battery Commander with 18th Airborne Corp Artillery in support of the 82nd Airborne Division. We were the lead assault force into the region during Desert Shield/Storm in 1990/1991. We had arrived in-country mid August, and had spent quite a bit of time just learning how to do extremely complicated things like figuring out how to breathe in 125 degree temperatures, as well as how to use the toilets in the Middle East. By late November we had figured it out.

We were dug into a canyon in front of a huge valley on the Iraqi/Saudi border (some said we were actually in Iraq, our maps left much to be desired), in what I felt was a standoff of Biblical proportions. We could see the enemy positions across the way along the escarpment on the other side of the valley and were actually firing on them every night. We were anticipating a huge battle and I had slowly but surely came to the realization that there was a distinct possibility that I might die during it. What I didn't realize at the time was, the war in the Desert wasn't actually the war I was going to eventually have to fight and win. Ultimately that war was the internal struggle to be the "real " (authentic) me.

One thing I enjoyed the most about being in this harsh place was how beautiful the stars were in the desert sky at night. It seemed like you could see for thousands of miles. On this particular evening I suddenly had a horrible revelation. While watching this beautiful display, I woke up to the fact that - **SHIT! I WASN'T LIVING THE "RIGHT" LIFE,** the life I was destined to be living.

I had this weird feeling like my life wasn't real, as if was like an old western town; with building facades that looked real but were actually just a front with nothing behind it. I hope none of you ever experience this feeling because it is really a bad feeling. I had struggled with being transgendered all my life but just felt like it was my "cross" to bear. In some morbid way I maybe even, on some level, hoped that I wouldn't make it back. However, that didn't happen, I SURVIVED! Yay? After that night though, I began to realize that I would have to start dealing with

20

this part of myself. I could not just keep pretending it was a bad habit or some weird game I was playing.

If you have ever been in the military, especially in times of war, you know you don't get many choices. You don't get to pick your outfit, what's for breakfast, what you're going to do today, and so on. I began to do something small in acknowledgment of this part of me. So I began to shave a spot on my leg. I couldn't control anything else but I could control that. This may not have been the wisest move because then body hair began to represent everything that was wrong with my body. I decided that I needed to start trying to figure this out so I wouldn't spend any more time than necessary living in the "wrong" gendered body.

We did, in fact, survive the war. I received many decorations including a Bronze Star. But all I was really thinking about was how I was going to be able to accomplish this seemingly impossible feat of getting to the right life for me. I knew the military was not going to be very excited about it. As I've learned throughout the years, once you decide you have something you need to do, the universe brings it about. The Army started downsizing, and I was offered an option to take an early release from active duty. I knew this feeling of wrongness from living with my male body wasn't going away, so I took the early release money and resigned my commission. It still took me 12 years to get myself into the right life. I was, however, finally on the road to getting there.

2. What was my life like "in the beginning"?

I had a relatively happy childhood. I spent the first 3 years (approximately) of my life on a farm in Minnesota. My Dad was a farmer and I eventually had 2 other sisters and was quite happy to be a part of this family. We moved into my little hometown of Windom, MN when I was about 3-4 years old. My first "real" memory was a bit traumatic. I was riding with my father to deliver our tractor to the implement dealer. It symbolized leaving the farm to me, which also left me with a life long love of farms and a vague sense of missing something.

I also felt very compelled to model my mother. She was always be trying to get me model my father but I was very determined to model her. This is one of the main discussion points of being transgendered. The question of "nature vs. nurture" -what causes this dilemma? I have never really considered this question. I have an Aunt who is a psychiatrist who casually mentioned this to my sister early in my transition and I pretty much laughed it off. I was

22

pretty resistant to any idea that was what I felt was "situational" or "socially" constructed. At this point in my life I'm now willing to admit that that anything is possible in the human experience.

At about 4 years of age an event happened which crystallized what "this" transgendered was, and how I was going to deal with it in the years to come. My mother caught me wearing my sisters' clothes in their closet (today we would say a child was "self expressing"). My mother made a point of embarrassing/shaming me before my sisters. At that point in time I like to say I went "underground". I realized that my family would not understand what it was that I struggled with, so hid "it" from everyone. I was, of course, afraid of being rejected by all those who were there to love and protect me. Nobody really wants to take that risk.

Today we read many stories about young transgendered kids who, for whatever reason, are able to articulate the distress of feeling incongruent in their own bodies.

I spent the next several years cross-dressing in private and hiding clothes in various hiding places throughout the home. Some would say I "compartmentalized" these feelings of mine. The only time I came close to being caught was by my father at around 9 or 10 years old. My father came up to get me and I had locked and put a chair under the door, and fortunately, I was able to get changed quickly enough that he didn't catch me.

My biggest crisis happened at puberty. My body began to change in ways I felt were wrong and this caused great anxiety for me. My older sister at one point came down into our basement, rubbed her hand on my leg and stated, "You're getting so hairy!" I really freaked out and actually went up and shaved the tops of my legs I was so distressed. Naturally I thought the whole world would realize I had done that, however, no one ever did and I didn't shave anything again until almost 20 years later.

My high school years were great. I like to say I had the perfect costume for hiding who I was. I went to a small school so I could be a musician and an athlete. I lettered in Football and Track and earned some distinction both as an athlete and as a musician. This is the only time of my life that I felt that my "inner female" was silent. There were many reasons for that. Testosterone levels are the highest in young men during this time frame, I was also very busy, and I was sexually active. I did something called "transference" (which is becoming less and less common in transgendered people today).

Transference is where we get the "access" to what we feel we should have had from birth. One gets fulfillment from second hand experiencing what our sexual partner is experiencing.

At the end of high school I enlisted in the Navy. Because I had been sexually active I ended up getting my high school girlfriend (who I loved deeply) pregnant. Living in a small town is great but in these types of circumstances it wasn't really where I wanted to live so we decided to get married and go where the Navy sent us.

Its important to note that at this time in my life I still did not understand what it was that I struggled with. I deeply loved my wife and never dreamed that I would want or need to be able to change my gender, so I just simply tried to live my life the best I could. I do think that one of my subconscious reasons for going in the service was to limit my interactions with women. One of my "flawed" reasons for believing that I felt like a woman was because I was around women too much. I know today this is not true but I had nothing else to go on, so in that circumstance our minds tend to jump to any conclusion that seems to make sense.

I spent the next 4 years in the Navy, got out and went to college, and then within 6 months went back in the Army as a commissioned officer. This was really the best option at the time for my family, but I believe that I also had a bit of a death wish, hoping that I would never have to deal with the reality of changing my gender. I almost got my wish.

After this realization in the desert, I knew I had to change my life, so I did. From the time I made this decision, to actually taking action, was a period of almost 8 years. Once the human mind conceives a plan the thoughts begin to change reality, both "actual" and "psychologically." When I decided to solve my dilemma the answers began to appear and take form and I began to know deep in my soul that eventually I would get to where I needed to go, to actually become a woman.

And now, after numerous years of speaking at colleges and miscellaneous groups, here are my answers to some of the interesting questions I have been asked over the years in regards to my life and transition to being a woman.

CHAPTER Two: The identity Alphabet Soup (Understanding the Difference between sex, sexuality, and gender).

3. What do LGBTQ Stand For?

L – Stands for Lesbian or female-to-female attraction.

G - Stands for Gay or male-to-male attraction.

B – Stands for Bisexual; someone who is, or can be, sexually attracted to both the same sex and the opposite sex.

T – Stands for Transgendered. It's interesting to note the difference here. The previous categories are all based on sexual attraction. Transgender, on the other hand, is about what gender someone identifies as.

Q – Stands for Queer or Questioning. Sometimes the terms "homosexual" or "heterosexual", or even "transgendered" are just too black and white. The grayness of Q helps people identify when they don't fit any of the other boxes that we as a society tend to put people into.

4. What does transgendered mean?

Transgendered simply refers to someone who is not comfortable with his or her own gender, or feels like they have been born in the wrong gender. There is a new term being used these days called "cisgendered." This is someone who is simply comfortable with the gender they are born with. Being transgender is not to be confused with a person's sexuality or whom they are sexually attracted to.

5. Why are some people transgendered?

There are a number of theories about why transgender people exist although there is not yet a scientific consensus.

When you look across cultures, you will find that people have had a wide range of beliefs about gender. Some cultures look at people and see six genders, while others see two. Some cultures have created specific ways for people to live in roles that are different from that assigned to them at birth. In addition, different cultures also vary in their definitions of masculine and feminine. Whether we view someone as transgender depends on the cultural lenses we are looking through as well as how people identify themselves.

Biologists tell us that sex is a complicated matter, much more complex than what we may have been taught in school. People who have XX chromosomes are generally considered female, while a person with XY chromosome is generally considered male. However, there are many people with XXY, XYY, and other variations of chromosomes; these genetic differences may or may not be visibly apparent or known to the person.

Some people are born with XY chromosomes, but are unable to respond to testosterone and therefore develop bodies with a vagina and breast, rather than a penis and testes. A variation in gender may just be a part of the natural order and there are more varieties than we generally realize. People with biological differences in gender may be considered intersexed; they may or may not self-identify as transgender.

There are many medical theories about why people are transgender. Some speculate that fluctuations or imbalances in hormones or the use of certain medications during pregnancy may cause intersexed or transgender conditions. Other research indicates that there are links between transgender identity and brain structure.

Some people believe that psychological factors are the reason for the existence of transgender people. It is clear that there are people who are aware that they are transgender from their earliest memories. Many transgendered people feel their gender identity is an innate part of them, an integral part of who they were born to be. Conversely, there are people who feel that everyone has a right to choose whatever gender presentation feels best or right to that individual. People should have the freedom to express themselves in whatever way is right for them.

Sex and gender are complex issues. A huge variety of factors are at work in making each individual the person that they are and there is no one reason that causes people to be transgender. Transgendered people are part of the variety that makes up the human community.

6. What is the difference between gender identity and sexual orientation?

Transgendered people may identify as heterosexual, lesbian, gay, or bisexual. The confusion comes into play when we perceive another as one gender and that doesn't match with how that person identifies with regards to sexual identity. Whether caused by a complication at birth, hormonal imbalances during puberty, irregular chromosomal make-up conflicting with fertility, or navigating impending menopause – gender, sex, and sexual identity are characteristics we all have and we all have to figure out about others and ourselves.

Think about surveys, which ask the demographic data of folks. Many people use Sex and Gender as synonyms, but they are actually very different. For the sake of this conversation, let's separate the two. Then we have Sexual Identity. I use the term Sexual Identity instead of Sexual Orientation as it seems to me to be a more inclusive way to describe who someone is romantically or sexually attracted to; that one's label to describe who they are attracted to may change as identifying language becomes known, or as you meet new people that challenge your Sexual Orientation to grow in new directions. An example of this is when a transgender person experiences a shift in who they are attracted to; a male to female transgendered person may begin to be attracted males even though they may have never been attracted before.

The whole discussion becomes more complicated as individuals transition, and to what extent one transitions. There are some who say that a completely transitioned MTF (male to female) is now a woman and if she is sexually with a woman, well then that's gay (lesbian). Some say because we are genetically still male (more and more a point of controversy), then if they are sexually with a man, well that's gay. This same logic applies to the FTM equation as well. Personally, I'm bisexual, so it really doesn't matter to me. However, as a male I was "not" attracted to men. Which brings up the issue that sometimes during transition sexual attraction actually changes and shifts. We have been schooled or trained to think that attraction is something intransient when in fact under the right circumstances things could, and in fact do, sometimes change.

7. Is gender identity the same as sex?

No. These are two separate issues. "Sex" in this sense usually implies biological body type i.e. male and female, and refers to biological differences; chromosomes, hormonal profiles, internal and external sex organs.

Gender identity is more fluid. This term refers to masculine or feminine energy and describes the characteristics that a society or culture delineates as masculine or feminine, which associations, I might add, vary widely around the world.

8. Can people overcome or be "cured" of being Gay or transgendered?

Simple answer... You can't, it's beyond your power.

It's the same as being black or white or having blue eyes or brown eyes.

It's not something you asked for, it's there, whether or you like it or not.

It's not a sin or a curse (unless you make it one).

The only thing you can do is make the best of it.

I do believe that you can manage to have a good life without fighting against yourself, 'cause that what it is, a part of you.

In most aspects of life, we are rewarded with fighting hard and not giving up. Unfortunately, many of us fight our own Gender and/or Sexual Identity with everything we have. We end up creating a faux or inauthentic life with spouses, children, lots of friends, and careers, simply because we are not living up to whom we perceive ourselves to be. At some point we hit a wall (age 44 for me) and GID (Gender Identity Disorder) demands your full attention and will not be ignored. If you have a little more strength to fight it, you can get by a little longer but the

33

GID will just increase and match your will to fight it. It will invade every thought and moment of your life so that you can't deal with anything else until you deal with IT.

My counselor at one point said that transgendered individuals should be applauded as we fight all of our lives to be who society expects us to be until we can't fight anymore. We become exhausted from the fight to be something that we just are not, and from literally living in two different worlds.

9. What are some categories of transgendered people, and what are their characteristics?

There used to be fewer definitive and more restrictive categories of transgendered persons. This has changed over the past 20 years and has evolved into the following categories*:

Intersexed: is a variation in sex characteristics including chromosomes, gonads, and genitals, seen in both humans and other animals, that do not allow an individual to be distinctly identified as male or female. Such variation may involve genital ambiguity, and combinations of chromosomal genotype and sexual phenotype other than XY-male, hermaphrodites, and XX-female. Intersex infants with ambiguous outer genitalia may be surgically 'corrected' to more easily fit into a socially accepted sex category. It is also sometimes referred to as a DSD or Developmental Sexual Disorder.

Bigender: A person who identifies as both genders.

Agender: A person who identifies as no gender.

Genderfluid: A person who is constantly moving between genders.

Third Gender/Third Sex: A person who does not identify as either male or female.

Genderqueer: A person who identifies as something other than just male or female. (Third Gender, Agender, Bigender, etc.)

Androgyne: A person who is neither feminine nor masculine, and doesn't identify with any gender.

Transvestite/Crossdresser: A person who wears clothing traditionally associated with the opposite sex.

Bio: A slang used in LGBT and butch and femme communities to describe a young person who looks and acts like a young, heterosexual male or female.

*Terms tend to be fluid and are constantly evolving, as we grow to understand all parts of ourselves better.

10. What is GID (Gender Identity Disorder)?

Gender identity disorder (GID), or transsexualism, is defined by strong, persistent feelings of self-identification with the opposite gender, and discomfort with one's own assigned sex. People with GID desire to live as members of the opposite sex and often dress and use mannerisms associated with the other gender. For instance, a person identified as a boy may feel and act like a girl. This is distinct from homosexuality in that homosexuals nearly always identify with their apparent sex or gender.

Identity issues may manifest in a variety of different ways. For example, some people with normal genitals and secondary sex characteristics of one gender privately identify more with the other gender. Some may cross-dress, and some may actually seek sex-change surgery. Others are born with ambiguous genitalia or chromosomes, which can also raise identity issues.

11. Is the trans community disproportionately affected by HIV/AIDS?

Depending on the study, transgendered people can be up to 4X more likely to be affected by HIV/AIDS. A recent Huffington Post article claims that transgendered women can be up 49 times more likely to have HIV/AIDS compared to the rest of society.

Now for a reality check: First of all HIV/AIDS is more affected by "what you do, as opposed to who you are". Secondly, HIV/AIDS is not a "gay" disease. It affects all spectrums of society. Thirdly, HIV/AIDS are two separate things. HIV is the inability of the white blood cells to multiply and reproduce. AIDS is any disease that cannot be fought because of a compromised immune system caused by HIV. Current medication allows the management of the disease from being actualized. Many individuals are now living with the disease and are managing well. HIV/AIDS are transmitted through blood-to-blood transmission anywhere in or on the body. Again, the most important thing to note is that HIV/AIDS is affected by "what you do" compared to "who you are". This means that a rather large number of trans women around the world survive by doing "at risk" activities like prostitution. I do not mean to imply that the majority of transgendered women are prostitutes, just that in third world countries without much other economic opportunities, this tends to be what happens. We all deserve to live, and if that is how they can survive I don't think the world should look down on them.

Other challenges to the collection of true statistics arise because of difficulties with reporting HIV/AIDS. Some transgender people may not identify as transgender due to fear of discrimination or previous negative experiences. Since some people in this community do not self-identify as transgender, relying solely upon gender to identify transgender people is not enough. Gender expression may fluctuate for some transgender people due to issues such as perceived safety or reluctance to identify as transgender in certain situations.

The Institute of Medicine has recommended that behavioral and surveillance data for transgender men and women should be collected and analyzed separately and not grouped with data for men who have sex with men. Using the 2-step data collection method of asking for sex assigned at birth and current gender identity increases the likelihood that all transgender people will be accurately identified in such studies.

12. What's the difference between a transgendered and a cross dresser, a transvestite, or a drag queen?

This is a rather complex question. There is some overlap between the groups. A cross-dresser and transvestite are similar although cross-dresser is many times a more "politically correct" term than transvestite. I will make an attempt to clarify.

Cross-dresser is a term many transgendered individuals prefer because it is simply the way a transgendered individual can propitiate how they feel inside themselves. There is also a category of cross-dresser (or transvestite) that is not transgendered.
For some there is a sexual component to cross-dressing it is exciting and non-conforming, which they find arousing. The transgendered community sometimes views this form of cross-dressing quite negatively. They want people to understand, at least for them, there is no sexual component to cross-dressing.

There is also a type of cross-dresser referred to as Drag Queens. Some drag queens emulate women, and some mock women. Most are usually Gay men but I have a good friend who did it because she was transgendered. In short, cross-dressing is not a "one size fits all" term!

13. Are there tests to determine if a person is transgendered?

General consensus is that being transgendered is a self-diagnosed disorder, however, there is a psychological test called the C.O.G.I.A.T.I. (Combined Gender Identity And Transsexuality Inventory) developed by Jennifer Diane Reitz. This test was "designed specifically for the uncertain pre-transitional Male-to-Female gender dysphoric individual", and might not make sense if you are otherwise.

Although no one test can determine with certainty if someone is a transgendered or not, by taking the test and then considering whether you agree or disagree with the results, and why, you might learn something about yourself. The hardest thing about this test is answering the questions honestly... it can be very hard to be honest with yourself.

14. What is autogynephilia?

Autogynephilia is the "mental illness" described by the pseudoscientific theory that male-to-female transsexuals who
aren't exclusively attracted to men actually have a sexual fetish for viewing themselves as females. This covers lesbian, bisexual, and pansexual transsexuals. The term translates from Greek to something like "self-woman-love," with the intended meaning "love of oneself as a woman." The theory was originated by Ray Blanchard and Kurt Freund in the 1980s, and endorsed by onetime celebrity psychologist J. Michael Bailey (who was later forced to resign as psychology chair at Northwestern University because of the controversy).

The theory is often accompanied by the notion that transsexuals attracted exclusively to men take an identical developmental route as homosexuals, but are so overtly effeminate that they find it difficult to operate in life as even a homosexual man. And since these transsexuals are developmentally identical to homosexual men, they are labeled "homosexual transsexuals." (Never mind that transsexuals describe their sexual orientation in terms of their preferred sex gender, meaning that trans women attracted to men consider themselves heterosexual.)

If you noticed something odd in the previous paragraphs, in that nothing in it can be meaningfully applied to female-to-male transsexuals, then you're absolutely right. That is because this theory completely ignores their existence.

This "theory has basically been disproven because so much of its assumptions are false. This resembles research bias; when someone makes a decision about something being true. They then find the specific facts that support their belief, and eventually after researching they pronounce their theory fact.

Some transgendered individuals do describe physical arousal as a part of cross-dressing, myself included. In my case, this arousal had nothing to do with who I was attracted to, but was, I believe, the euphoria of being able to express myself as my authentic self.

15. Why can't you just stop doing this (cross-dressing, etc...)?

I believe it's simply because it is who we are. Many transgendered people go through what we call "purges", where we throw away our female wardrobe. However, you cannot just throw parts of yourself away, and that is essentially what they are attempting. Cross-dressing is simply the manifestation of this repressed part of who we are. I spent a significant amount of time trying to understand why I was so compelled to dress like a woman. It took me almost 30 years to be able to truly face myself, and that is not an unusual amount of time.

16. Do people transition to get away from personal problems?

I don't think people exclusively do it for this reason. I have met some people who I felt like they just didn't like who they were and were trying to get away from "who" they were. We like to say, "If you were an a-hole as a man then you will probably be a bitch on the other side." I think this is too simple of an answer. There is a significant amount of self-hatred associated with being transgendered, and if someone has incorporated so much of this into their psyche then there is much more personal work that needs to be done.

17. Did I transition because I was so freaked out about being gay?

This is one of the more interesting questions I've been asked. I believe this is a commonly held belief among a certain group of people (who are probably homophobic to some extent). I had a funny talk with my youngest son a couple of years ago. He was complaining about not understanding his wife, and women in general and how confusing they were, and then he made the comment, "Sometimes I wish I was gay!" I had this epiphany moment and looked at him and said, "ME TOO." It would have been so much easier.

Really! The whole journey for a gay person is coming to the conclusion that they are, well, gay. They don't change their bodies. For us, accepting being transgendered is just the beginning of a long and potentially painful journey. So I did not transition so I could have "sex" with guys, which, by the way, is probably the underlying issue for the previously mentioned people. That being said, when I was dealing with my gender identity before transitioning, I just simply was never attracted sexually or otherwise, to men, which, by the way, is the number one factor of being gay. I *would* occasionally have the thought, "am I

44

gay?" But then I would remember that I wasn't wired that way.

I have been in long-term relationships with men at this point in my life and I enjoy men, but I am still visually attracted to women, (they wear brighter colors, they take pride in their appearances) so now I consider myself bisexual. Ain't life weird? I have had brief relationships, which, by the way, I thoroughly enjoyed, but no long-term relationships with women since transitioning.

18. Are transgendered people Gay?

This is a question that gets asked quite bit. There is generally significant confusion about sex and gender. A transgendered individual's internal conflict with their body revolves around gender, not sex. When questioned why are we grouped in with the GBL community I like to say we just get beat up by the same people, which is sadly true.

Many times a person transitions into their correct gender and who they are attracted to changes. Many times it does not. Most experts say 33% of the time it stays the same, 33% of the time it changes, and 33% of the time people just stay confused.   It's a bit complicated because there can be other factors at play.

In my case, as a guy I was never attracted to guys. I was very attracted to women. As I began to transition a strange thing happened and I found myself being attracted to guys. No one can really explain why some transgendered individual's attraction changes. Some attribute it to the hormones; some attribute it to "latent" gay tendencies. In my case it just naturally occurred.

Since completing my transition, I have been in long-term relationships with men. I am still very attracted to women, and consider myself bi-sexual now.   This became clearer to me while speaking to a college class once. I did my usual talk about how it worked for me and then one guy in the back of the room spoke up and asked me, "so as you look out on us, who catches your eye?"   It was absolutely without question the women that caught my eye.

However, as I talked and thought about the subject I realized it was their clothes and accessories that I was checking out.   There wasn't anything sexual about why I was drawn to women, I was just admiring their outfits. It is sometimes more complicated than that, and I have still sometimes been attracted to, and have had brief sexual or romantic relationships with, women since transitioning.

19. Do people transition for sex?

Early in my transition I would get this question. I was very much trying to help people understand the difference between sex, sexuality, and gender identity. I would sometimes react with quite a bit of anger toward this question. I had not figured out my own sexuality at that point. So far I have never met anyone who openly did this for sex, but I don't rule it out. I think as a society we are very insecure about our individual sexuality. I used to feel very strongly, especially when I was struggling with the overall issue. Thinking that I would not transition if it were about sexuality. I have become so much more comfortable with my sexuality that I have now backed away from this judgment.

20. ...Is "it" contagious?

Yes, I've actually been asked that! But NO it is not. This is another myth that some people like to perpetuate. My oldest son has 3 sons and this was one of their concerns about my transition. If people are open to information (as my son and his wife were) this can be quickly dispensed with. If there is any contagion, it is that by our being open with our families and friends, it gives others the courage to follow their own hearts.

I have a rather funny story relating to this. Sometime after we had worked through some of the initial problems, occasionally our family would go out to eat after church. My oldest grandson was about 6 years old; we finished eating and decided to go the bathroom together. He finished and then came out and was yelling into the women's bathroom, "Hey Papa, what are you doing in the Ladies' room? You're not a lady!"

One of the things we like to do with children is to honestly answer their questions while not overloading them with information. So we went outside and had a little talk about how when I was a little boy my head told me I was a girl. After finishing my story I looked at him and he was standing with a little frown on his face. He then looked at me and said, "Sometimes my brain tells me I'm a girl, but I just tell it I'm a boy and to shut up." One thing I'd forgotten about kids was that they are great empathizers, but I had quite a shock until I figured that out.

21. How does someone know if they are transgendered?

This is hard to describe because it is still something that is referred to being a "self-diagnosed" condition. There are no blood tests or any other kinds of tests that can clearly state that someone is this way. I like to say it is a spirit or soul condition. Most (75%) of the transgendered individuals I've met said they had known at very early ages that they are transgendered. There are some that come to a realization later, but, in general, as little children become self aware they realize they are different than what their families think they are. I've read that as soon as kids can talk they say things like, "Mommy, I'm a boy," or "I'm a girl."

22. Do all transgendered individuals have surgery to change their gender?

Studies indicated only about 20% of MTF and only about 3-5% of FTM actually have surgery. Most of the surgery is not covered by insurance, which makes it a pretty large financial hurdle for most individuals. Some larger companies like Intel are starting to cover it, but overall most insurance plans do not cover it, yet. It is my belief that the younger generations are becoming more and more comfortable with being an "in between" gender. I am a little older and probably more conventional so I could not envision doing the transition without surgery. At this point I'm not clear on exactly how the culture and generational differences have driven me in this decision, but I'm sure if I looked deep enough I'd find the reasons.

CHAPTER Three: The Inner Struggle/Emotional Life of Being Transgendered.

23. Is being transgendered a mental disorder? And if yes is it curable?

There is considerable discussion on this topic. The old title was "gender identity disorder" or GID. The new DSM-5 classifies this as "gender dysphoria" which focuses more attention on those who feel distressed by their gender identity. This is a small reduction in the stigma attached to the old term. There is a move to remove the diagnosis altogether, just as homosexuality was removed from the DSM-4 in 1973. The logic behind leaving the diagnosis in is to ensure that a transgendered person can still access health care if needed, such as for hormone treatment or counseling for those that need help dealing with their emotions, and those that want to transition to their correct gender.

Unfortunately, in the old DSM-4 it was put in the same section as pedophilia (child molesters) and paraphilia, in a section called, sexual and gender disorders. With more and more information becoming available about transgenderism it has since been moved to a different section in the new DSM-5. However, because of the grouping in the old DSM, individuals with agendas (typically conservative religious types) like to make the leap that transgendered people are also child molesters. This has happened recently with Michelle Duggar on the reality series, "19 Kids and Counting." Sadly, ignorance and fear go hand in hand and hopefully one-day people will not fear others that are not like them.

My answer for the second part of this question is that, yes, in my opinion, it is curable. However, sometimes the cure is as painful as the "disease". In some cases, depending on how strong the need is, transition is typically the cure for this situation. I've known some who were able to live with and adapt to gender dsyphoria without changing their gender.

24. When did I know I was transgendered?

I knew very young that something was "different" about me. Most kids have childhood amnesia and don't really have many memories before the age of 3 or 4. That was true in my case. My first inklings were when my mom kept telling me to emulate my dad when I wanted to emulate her. Most kids go through a "puppy phase" where they follow a parent around and emulate them. I immediately identified with my mom rather than my Dad.

I did not actually know what I was; I just knew something was different. That was pounded home to me when I was 4 years old. I was dressing in my sisters' clothes in their closet, and my mom caught me and made a huge deal of it. She kept reminding everyone of this incident for the next 40 years. I would always think to myself, "if she only knew..." then one day she did. However, at 4 years old, the only thing I knew was that I couldn't share this secret desire with the most important people in my life, my family. I came to look at it like a game, sort of a secret spy thing, and that's how I dealt with it for most of my life.

25. Was I ever molested as a child and could that explain why you are transgendered?

I was raised in a small town with two sisters and a stay at home mom. I had a pretty ideal childhood at least with regards to this type of situation. I personally have no memories of ever being molested and am certain that this never happened to me.

There are many societal theories about what causes us to be transgendered. I have been asked if my mom was dominant and did that cause me to want to be a girl. Did she do something to me, sexually, that resulted in me being transgendered? Some moms even feel guilt about a transgendered child. Did they do something when they were pregnant that cause this to occur? My mom was no different, she felt like she had somehow failed me. We had a very poignant talk at one point and I had to reassure her that nothing she did caused this to happen.

As more and more transgendered kids speak up and tell us how they want to present their individuality in our world, this question becomes more and more irrelevant. Most of them just want to be able to live and express exactly who and what they are. This is usually expressed through what they want to wear, toys they want to play with, etc. As more and more light is shed on trans kids we are seeing more and more that this is how they "feel" or how they see themselves, and they don't necessarily self-identify with who or what their world sees them as.

All that being said, I have also heard of some unusual situations where someone is criticized for something like the size of their penis, or that they are so pretty. These people have sometimes been told things like this since they were small. In general, being transgendered is a self-diagnosed condition. However, some professional counselors will say that if someone is told something repeatedly throughout their childhood, that they will sometimes incorporate that belief into their psyche. This is rare but it does happen occasionally. I've heard of people getting all the way to the surgeons table before coming to the realization that this is not who they are. This is a big reason for why we have counselors involved in our transitions.

26. Describe the thought process during the time I was struggling with this?

My thoughts were continuously on, thinking about how wrong my life was. It's similar to when you are attracted to someone and they occupy your thinking no matter how hard you try to get them out of your head. I suppose you could say at this point in my life I was insanely in love with...well...myself. I actually thought I would go insane if I didn't do something about it, it was like slowly driving me mad. Once I began to commit to this journey I began to slowly feel sane again. Sometimes people ask why I would choose this "lifestyle." I tell them that I literally was unable to continue on the road I was on. I sincerely believe I would have died either figuratively or literally if I was unable to solve this dilemma in my life.

Sometimes I felt like it was a "sin." I had heard a definition of sin many years ago that basically resonated with me which said, "What got in the way of my relationship with God, was...sin." Because I felt that this was in the way of my relationship with God I assumed being transgendered was a sin. I now believe "God" loves all of us unconditionally and, really, the concept of a benevolent "God" who is "out there" is not really how I believe the universe is put together.

27. What role does depression and anxiety play in transitioning?

The prevalence of depression and anxiety amongst the trans communities is higher than for other lesbian, gay and bisexual people.

In an Australian survey of LGBT people, around 60% of transgender males and 50% of transgender females reported having depression. A 2007 survey of Australian and New Zealand transgender people found that almost 90% had experienced at least one form of stigma or discrimination, including verbal abuse, social exclusion, receiving worse treatment due to their name or sex on documents, physical threats and violence. Almost two thirds of participants reported modifying their activities due to fear of stigma or discrimination. People experiencing a greater number of different types of discrimination were more likely to report being currently depressed.

In general, the majority of lesbian, gay, bi, trans and intersexed (LGBTI) people lead happy, healthy, fulfilling lives. However, studies have found that non-heterosexual people face up to twice as much abuse or violence (including physical, mental, sexual or emotional) than their heterosexual counterparts. This prejudice and discrimination adds an additional layer of risk on top of biological, social, environmental and psychological factors, which can lead to depression and anxiety.

Research and real life experiences have found that LGBT people have an increased risk of depression and anxiety, substance abuse, and self-harming behavior, as well as suicidal thoughts.

When compared with heterosexual people, homosexual and bisexual people are twice as likely experience anxiety (31.5% compared with 14.1%) and three times as likely to experience depression and related disorders (19% compared with 6%).

My experience was mainly with anxiety. Once I made the decision to transition, if I felt blocked or felt like I was not progressing on my journey I would feel tremendous anxiety, even panic. I have many transgendered friends that deal with tremendous depression. I've also had two intimate partners commit suicide, so these statistics hit close to home.

28. Is it typical for transgendered individuals to be addicts?

It is estimated that 30 percent of the LGBT population struggles with some form of addiction; whether drugs, alcohol, sex or gambling. Contrast that figure with the approximately 9 percent of the general population is impacted by addiction and it's not hard to see that addiction is an epidemic in the LGBT community.

Nowhere is this more prevalent that in the transgender community where rates of addiction tend to be even higher. While most addiction research has focused largely on gay men and lesbians, and less so the bisexual community, it's important to put equally as much focus on the transgender community.

According to a Substance Abuse and Mental Health Services Administration (SAMHSA) study, "The stress that comes from daily battles with discrimination and stigma is a principal driver of these higher rates of substance use, as transgender people turn to tobacco, alcohol, prescription drugs, and other substances as a way to cope with these challenges." "Transgender people face disproportionate levels of stress, due to social prejudice and discriminatory laws," say advocates. This can result in increased anxiety, depression and isolation, leading many to self-medicate with illegal or prescription drugs, or alcohol. Also, many trans people find a safe space in the bar or club scene, again increasing exposure to alcohol and drugs.

29. What are the most important personal tools and characteristics that can assist someone going through this process?

Patience, confidence, and love for oneself (most people can be self-loathing), love for others, patience for others, being able to see yourself as your desired man/woman, flexibility, staying connected (as much as possible) with your family and friends, and staying optimistic.

CHAPTER Four:
Spirituality/Religion/Philosophical issues

30. Have transgendered people always existed or is this a new phenomenon?

The oldest theorized transgender person dates to around 2500 B.C. in the Czech Republic. The body that archeologists unearthed was buried in a manner designed for women of that time period, but was examined and conclusively determined to be the skeleton of a male.

Scientists who worked on this project concluded that the remains were likely those of a transgender person, although it has also been suggested that it is possible that the grave is that of a gay man. Unfortunately, these two ideas have become crossed over and articles refer to the potential transgenderism of this person as their sexual identity when it is not. Regardless, this *may* be the oldest known transgender person.

There are references in the bible to "eunuchs," who, some speculate, were transgendered persons. Matthew 19:12 make reference to what Jesus had to say. Paraphrasing, he said that those who are "born that way" should live that way. In certain cultures, the term "eunuch" refers to asexual people, while in others it refers to males whose testicles were removed in childhood, leading to development without testosterone, which may have caused transgender-like symptoms that we nowadays induce by introducing estrogen to the male body.

Transgender people are known to have existed throughout almost all of recorded history, including back to very early civilizations in places like Europe, the Middle East, and even the Americas, where they are well documented among Native American tribes and are known as Two-Spirit people.

In nearly all cultures where transgender people are known to have existed, they were typically treated with high regard and believed to be more knowledgeable than a cisgendered person (a person born with a gender identity that matches their physical body). Transgender people were often put into important positions within the religions of any given culture. In most of these cultures, male-to-female (MTF) people are often given higher recognition despite the fact that female-to-male (FTM) people also existed. These is largely because women were used in many religious ceremonies and were the ones thought to be able to commune with deities of their time.

Coupled with being recognized as women and believed to possess higher knowledge, these MTF people were quite revered in many cultures. FTM people were also recognized as men and took on traditional male roles within their society. However, as time passed and civilizations began to develop, the rise of patriarchy threatened transgender people a great deal, largely because they were believed to have special knowledge and male leaders began to fear this. In time, transgender people became repressed in many societies, although matriarchal societies continued to maintain their views, as did the Native American cultures.

31. What does the Bible have to say about all of this? Isn't this like mutilation or something?

I always love these questions. For many years I considered myself a born again Christian, and so I can empathize. The main verses that get pointed out to me are Deuteronomy 22:5, which states, "a man shall not dress as a woman", the problem with this verse is that the next verse, 22: 6 states, "and a woman shall not dress like a man." Anyone can tell that this verse is more of cultural thing rather than some kind of law. We know that cultural norms have definitely changed over the centuries. Most Christian religious images portray Jesus and the disciples wearing garments that look quite a bit like simple modern dresses that woman wear today. Do we even know what men and women wore back in the Old Testament times? Seems like an extremely vague law to try and enforce.

The most appropriate verse that I have ever found is in the book of John 1:1, verses 5-7, it is included in virtually all translations of the Bible. This verse makes a comment about having a "shadow" self. It goes on to say that it is "bad" to have a shadow self it very important to live a "shadowless" life. It also talks about doing whatever it takes to "not" have a shadow self. For many years that is how I perceived this side of myself, like a shadow of how I am supposed to be living this life.

As far as the mutilation part of this question, many transgendered people think of being transgendered as a "birth defect." As a society we condone the fixing of babies born with cleft palates, we repair babies that are born with an exposed heart, we separate conjoined twins, and the list goes on. According to this question all of these should be considered "mutilations" as well. This doesn't even go into the babies that are born intersexed and doctors making arbitrary decisions about their gender at the moment of birth rather than waiting until they grow up and tell their parents which gender they are. I personally know of a little boy that was born with both a penis and a vagina. The doctors sewed up the vagina and proclaimed he was a "boy." I met this little boy at a church that I was the worship leader for. His mother told me about what had happened. She was distressed about it and wondered if it had been the "right" decision.

This doesn't even begin to go into all the other human biological abnormalities that occur around the world. There are no clear statistics on how often these things occur, some estimate it is as common as someone being born with red hair or green eyes. The biological term for babies born with gender abnormalities is Disorder of Sexual Development or DSD. These can range from ambiguous genitalia to babies born with fully developed genitalia of both genders. Again this is just the "biological" issue. If you factor in all the psychological, emotional, and spiritual issues this "disorder" becomes extremely complex. The best advice is allowing them to grow up and tell the world who they are, rather than arbitrarily making them into what we think they are.

Just a personal note here: I believe the great fear of parents and even individuals is that no one will love them if they have unusual genitalia or if they are transgendered. The studies that have been made, and my own life experience, have found that people *do not* fall in love with genitalia but rather with our souls. This fear tends to be greatly exaggerated.

32. What is unique about being transgendered, and how is it similar to other struggles that human beings go through?

Being transgendered is unique, just as everything we experience as human beings is unique. It is more "in your face" and public than many of the other unlimited experiences we have as human beings. It is also unique in that it deals with sexuality in an unconventional way. Many people are pretty rigid in their views of sexuality, and so it is sometimes difficult to reach them, or ever really explain things like this, because they are closed to hearing anything outside of the norm. It is similar to other struggles that we have as human beings, because we each in our own way, *do* struggle with it. After I tell my story, many people tell me about themselves and what they've had to struggle with in life. I believe we are all- or at least we should be- trying to be authentic in who we are. In some ways we are some of the most authentic people on the planet. That can also be troubling to some people who are having difficulty finding their own authentic selves. Most people "hide" their true selves, whatever that means, from everyone in their world. I think that those who have chosen to transition are simply more transparent than most people.

33. If you could have been born a woman, would you have done that?

Yes. There are certain events that I never got to experience, like bearing a child. Many of the things that I learned growing up as a boy have served me well after my transition, however, so it's also made me somewhat unique and unusual, according to some women. Amazingly, the major difference is that I display much more confidence than the typical woman. Most women are not socialized to be confident, but rather to acquiesce to men. This occasionally results in me sticking out when I'm in a group of women.

The flip side to this question is, "if I could have been born a man without the conflict, would I have chosen that?" The answer to this question is once again yes. However, at this point it gets a little ridiculous, and we can get into a whole different discussion of "if not this, then what?" I believe that everyone on the planet gets something, some challenge that each one has to overcome, and this question denies this truth.

CHAPTER Five: Transitioning With Family & Friends

34. How could you do this to your family and embarrass or hurt them like this?

The presumption is that we are embarrassing our families. Some people do see this as an embarrassment, and disown and even disinherit the family member that's choosing to transition. I find that very sad and even inhumane. We are simply trying to be the best and most authentic human being we can be, and, I might add, stay alive in the process. So many individuals get to the end of their lives and feel like we have missed something important - this was not something I wanted to feel at my end.

Short of doing something traumatic, like transitioning, family and societal fears tend to keep us feeling trapped, while threats of abandonment keep us quite literally trapped in our skins.

We all have something called a "sacred wound" in our lives. It's the one thing that everyone on the planet gets, and while it gives him or her the opportunity to become whom he or she are supposed to be, it is usually wrapped up in our greatest fear.

For some of us it is being transgendered. For others it might be being born without arms or legs. For others it might be some type of trauma that happens during our lives (rape, losing our sight or hearing, maybe becoming paralyzed). No one, in my opinion, gets off the planet without having to deal with his or her "sacred wound." Many people respond by avoiding whatever their wound is or (also quite common) becoming embittered by it. I believe that success in life is taking whatever that "wound" is and overcoming it and making it into the greatest strength in our lives.

35. Is this something that young children would emulate and/or model (is it contagious)?

One of the common myths about being transgendered is that it is a choice that we make. One's gender is inherently part of who they are. We now know that the primary sex organ in anyone's body is a their brain. It tells us who we are and more importantly, what we are. I can no more influence a child to become transgendered than I can convince them that they are a dog or cat. It just simply is not who or what they are. I think that the thing the kids should model and emulate about the transgender issue is our drive to be authentic and real human beings, to me that is a powerful thing to emulate. I've heard the LGBT community's response to this question as follows: "I grew up with two heterosexual parents as role models and they didn't influence me to be heterosexual, so how can I influence anyone to be something they are not?"

36. Did your family ever suspect what was going on with you?

When many transgendered people tell their families, they are surprised to learn that their families had known for years. The so-called puzzle pieces just all came together. This isn't always the case. Almost none of my family ever guessed it. I had such a "big man" smoke screen going that most were pretty dumbfounded. I had told my youngest sister a few years before anyone else, and then my daughter, but other than that, no one else knew. You see, one of the biggest issues with coming out as being transgendered is the incredible fear that the people closest to you will reject you. This is a very effective jailer for most people. No one wants to be rejected or even ridiculed by his or her families.

37. What did your parents say?

I told my mother about a year before I told my dad. My mother had a classic feminine response. She said, "I don't know what transgendered means, but you are my child and I will always love you." I told my dad a year later and his comment was, and I quote, "why would anyone want to sit down to pee"? I found that very funny, and of course, why would anyone want to sit down to pee if they didn't have to? Men tend to see things from a practical perspective and that was my dad. My dad went on to become one of my greatest supporters. I overhead him at a family reunion a couple years before he died as he was talking to someone who was asking about me, and he said, "we don't throw kids away." If I hadn't really loved my dad before that I would have fallen in love with him all over again.

My mom developed Alzheimer's shortly after I transitioned and she always struggled with keeping it straight in her head. Some people in my family claimed her grief over my being transgendered and transitioning caused the onset of the disease, but I don't really think so. If it, in fact, had to do with grief, it started long before my transition. Grief is a strange thing. It has to be confronted eventually. Most people think they can bypass grief sometimes, but grieving has to ultimately happen. I believe that my mom did not grieve adequately for three stillborn babies earlier in her life, and before she could grieve for me she had to go back and grieve for them. I recall several conversations before the onset of Alzheimer's where she was crying and talking about the babies.

That being said, I know my parents did grieve for the person they thought I was. I was the only boy in our family and they did need to grieve for that. Some might find that strange but it is a very important aspect of the transition, especially among families.

Logically and biologically, I felt like I did my "duty" as the only son in my family, at least in respect to carrying on the family name. I have two sons who both have three sons. So one could say that I did carry out my responsibilities from some sort of biological standpoint. I am not saying that others should do that, it just seemed like I was supposed to carry on my family's name before I could transition to being a woman. This was never a huge concern for me, although it can be a concern in some families.

Eventually, my dad would come to always get my name right, although he would always say my male name first, and then correct himself. Both of my parents have passed on as of this writing but I will always be grateful to them for their love and acceptance.

38. What did your other siblings think?

I actually told my younger sister before anyone else. She had thought it a little strange when I was back for a family funeral and it appeared that I was shaving the hair off my body. After the funeral both of my sisters and I went out to a bar and after a couple of drinks we did a kind of thing where we dared each other to tell something about each that no one else knew. My older sister opted out but my younger sister was in.

After dropping off my older sister we went to the younger one's apartment and confided in each other.

I later told my older sister when I began transitioning. Her first comment was, "Can you not wait until our parents have passed away before you do this?" This is a comment I hear frequently from family members. The issue is, unfortunately, not just about the parents or family, but rather about the individual transitioning as well. Waiting was not an option at this point in my transition. My comment back to her was that I would probably beat them to the grave if I tried waiting. Change is uncomfortable no matter how it arrives in our lives and trying to accommodate others' fears and concerns begin to take second place to one's own needs and desires.

The other issue, with this community especially, is that the rate of suicide is extremely high. Many do take this route in order to spare their families the trauma of changing, unfortunately this route has a much more traumatic result. Most of us have put our families, friends, jobs, and more before our own needs for many years, and finally we just have to be who we are. The crises this causes in other peoples lives are, for the most part, their own expectation and reaction issues to deal with.

I believe there is a loving way to do this and a harsh way. Many things can be mitigated to smooth the transition, but ultimately the individual is compelled to change regardless of the others in their circles who want them to stay as they are.

39. How do you deal with siblings talking about your childhood?

This is one of the harder aspects of my relationship with my sisters. They like to talk to my kids about different things that happened during our childhood and inevitably it always comes up that they referred to me with the pronoun "he." When they first started doing this it made me very uncomfortable. I like to say, "it created a blip in my reality bubble," however, nowadays I feel like I have resolved my inner conflict around this issue and it is not been quite as much of a problem to deal with anymore. Ultimately, naturally I would not want to talk about my past because of this problem. I have no control of this, however, so I have to deal with it the best way I can. Sometimes I just excuse myself and sometimes my sisters do it when I'm not there. Sometimes I am just quiet and let them tell the story.

I think that it's hard for many people to talk about their past, not just transgendered people. Throughout our lives, we grow and change as humans on the planet; over time we move into different lives and become different people. Some people, and unfortunately this can be our family, can keep us trapped within their stories and beliefs about who we are. This is not to say that I am negating part of our lives; I'm just saying it isn't as relevant anymore.

Our past can become quite incongruent with who we are today, other than as a part of our story. I find it difficult at times to slip back and forth between two different stories. The other day my daughter brought up an instance with our family dog and how I was mean to the dog. I have a lot of guilt associated with how I treated that animal; and we talked about it and I said I would always regret how I treated that dog. We are all to some extent a product of our environment and of our upbringing. This doesn't necessarily have to control who we are today.

40. What do your kids call you?

Being a father was always very important to me. Most parents don't really think about the importance of being a parent when starting a family, but I very much love my kids and still feel some responsibility to make them happy. When I began this journey I really did not want my kids to have to change how they saw me and what they called me, thus I really wanted them to keep calling me Dad.

However, I got to a point in my transition to where that became increasingly uncomfortable to me and I felt myself unconsciously pulling away from them. It was after a group counseling session in which my whole family came and participated that I came to that realization. One of my daughter-in-laws pointed out that I was not congruent. She basically said she didn't see anything different.

After that I sat down with each of my kids and explained that I couldn't, at least for the foreseeable future have them call me Dad anymore. We came up with a compromise and that was to call me Dee. Dee could stand for DeAnna or Dad but it did not have the same "charge" as the term "Dad" did for me. Because of my long-term relationships it proved impossible to keep the "Dad" title. My grandkids and I did not share that kind of long- term relationship so I thought I could still have them call me Papa. This sort of worked until one day when I joined them at a local park. My grandsons started yelling at me, "Papa, papa!" As they did that, all the other kids playing on the playground looked up and were looking for a "papa." Shortly after that incident my oldest grandson thought maybe we should come up with a new name they could use as well. They came up with Dee Dee, and they all call me that now. My kids have also adopted the new name of Dee Dee.

Not all transgendered people have kids or grandkids. Many of them can easily continue to have their kids call them by their original family title. In my case when my kids called me "Dad," it would create a "blip" in my reality bubble, which was, in my case, very disconcerting. This can also become a problem if the family is not supportive of the transgendered individual; and can become a way of insulting them by using their former names, titles, and pronouns to humiliate them. I believe it is good to change these names and the titles, as that makes it easier to keep the pronouns correct as well. The solution, again, just depends on the individuals and their families.

41. Do you celebrate Father's Day?

We did celebrate it for a short period of time. Then, just like the Dad title becoming unsustainable for me, so did a national holiday dedicated to the old me. So, after I asked my kids to stop calling me "Dad" we decided that we should probably try something new. We picked a compromise of June 6 the actual "D Day." It was convenient because it actually falls between Mother's Day and Father's Day. We celebrated it for a couple of years and it was fun and novel. Then two of my grandkids were born right around that same time frame and instead of going back to Father's Day we have just kind of gently let it go. A small casualty of my transition I suppose you could say.

As mentioned in an earlier question, some individuals have no trouble keeping their same title, i.e. Dad. I have several friends who have their children continue to call them Dad (or Mom). However, I felt myself distancing myself from them when they used my old title. As they would call me Dad, a part of me would subconsciously try to "be Dad." I didn't realize it at first, but I was walking too fine of a line.

42. What do you think about kids that say they are transgendered?

We are seeing more media exposure about younger and younger kids who are self-identifying as the opposite gender. This has given much credence to our own stories, because most kids are not thought of as being sexual in any way, shape, or form. This either blows the myth that transsexuals change their gender because of sex, or the one that kids are non-sexual. Maybe both. You decide.

I knew I had the wrong body at about 3-4 years old. I also learned at 4 years old that I would be embarrassed because of it and in fact did get embarrassed by it. My mother caught me in my sister's closet, at the age of 4 years old, dressing in my sister's clothes. My mom told that story for years and years at practically every family reunion, which in some ways kept me in hiding for years.

It is very encouraging to hear story after story about these children facing up to their parents and describing themselves at being different than what their bodies look like. There is more information out about the whole transgendered dilemma; however, these kids don't necessarily have access to this information. Imagine my situation, where there was no information available and no one who understood what this was about.

I guess my "technique" was simply trying to survive and cope with a quite bewildering world. I think most kids in my generation would really not question what the parents were telling us, rather than believe our own internal cognitive understandings of who we are. I think if my parents would have asked the right questions at 4 years old I might have had a very different outcome. On the other hand I cannot be sure, it might have gotten much worse.

43. How do you deal with children?

Children are children. I've been told by any number of counselors to simply tell kids what they want to know. In other words, answer their questions honestly, and on the level that they can comprehend. Children, especially young ones, haven't developed the filters that adults have. They also tend to be curious and aren't shy about questioning what they see. That is amazing and problematic.

One time I had little boy follow me around when I was appraising a house. In the middle of talking about his toy he point blank asked me, "are you a boy or a lady?" I turned to him and said that I was a lady. He simply was confused, and, once I stated what I was, he was fine. I have another friend, who, while out shopping in a department store, was confronted by a little boy with the same question. He was a little more adventurous so he asked the little boy, "what do you think I am?"

The little boy looked at him for a while and then said, "I think you are a very pretty man." I have one grandson who holds me quite firmly to being a boy. He was at first quite threatened by me and would kind of badger me and ask me questions all the time. I was persistent as well, and eventually he has come to understand what it's about, at least from a seven-year-olds perspective.

44. Do you keep in touch with Army friends? High School friends?

I've lost touch with most of my Army friends, however, I have recently begun to establish connections with high school friends through Facebook. I actually ran into a woman, that I went to high school with, at the airport in Minneapolis. She walked right up to me, asked my name, and then hugged me, and I had no idea who she was. She turned out to be someone that I played next to in high school band. I have recently also connected with other friends I went to high school with, and I am expecting to go back to my high school reunion in the next year and reconnect with them.

CHAPTER Six: Transitioning (Before and After) With Sexual and/or Love Relationships.

45. Did Your Transition Cause Your Divorce?

In a word, yes. My wife actually was understanding and initially tried to stay but it was just too hard for her. My generation had little to no information about what being transgendered meant. Therefore, many of us just went ahead and lived our lives not really knowing what this would become. Many of us got married and had kids. As the Internet has become more available and accessible, many transgendered individuals have not gotten in relationships. Some marriages do survive the transition.

There are many variables, which can and do complicate staying in a relationship. Sometimes our attraction can change (mine did). A person can feel just as trapped as they had felt previously by being in the wrong body. Sometimes attraction stays the same and sometimes we become bi-sexual. Many women married to a transgendered partner want out because they did not sign up to be married to a woman and do not want to be in a "Lesbian" relationship. If women know upfront what they are getting into, there's a good chance it may survive. I've known couples that deeply love each other but tragically cannot deal with the gender change.

I've been asked, "Why did I get in a relationship, if I knew I would ultimately end up hurting that person?" I always ask the person if they had ever been hurt in a relationship, and whether or not that was their intent when the initially became involved. The answer of course is that no normal person would do that, but most of us have been hurt one time or another in a relationship. I also did not ever think this would ever manifest in the way that it has.

46. What do you tell people you date? Did that change pre-op and post-op?

The answer to this is a bit of a story. I have three transgender friends. One will not even meet someone that doesn't know all about her history. My second friend says that "kissing is just play," but before she would have sex with someone she would definitely tell them about her history. The third friend, after having sex with her boyfriend turns to him and says, "Babe we need to talk."

I always thought my third friend's story was the worst way to tell someone. However, I went on a date with a guy I met on-line once and ended up being totally honest and telling him about my past. Telling him pretty much ended the date. At that point though since he wasn't unfriendly and so I asked him what advice he had for someone like me, and he said, "maybe if you had really hot sex with him, maybe that would be enough to overlook the history." Well, at the time I thought that was the dumbest, not to mention scariest, thing I had ever heard! The point being that men do not like being surprised. Men tend to be slightly more homophobic than women. For example I had a friend of a friend living with me for a while and he actually picked up a prostitute and she turned out to be transgendered. She wouldn't get out of his car and so he pulled a baseball bat out of his trunk, and so yeah, *that* could have ended very badly.

The guideline I recommend to specifically transwomen who want to date men, but could apply to transmen wanting to date women, is that it takes some time to get to know someone. In our support group we kind of determined that 8 hours was an average amount of time that it takes to get to know anyone. Then we figured an average date goes about 3 hours. So we came up with the 3-date rule, before telling someone about being transgendered. If you don't have chemistry with someone anyway, what is the point of outing yourself?

Now today I participate in quite of bit of sacred sexuality workshops and events. I rarely tell anyone about myself because it puts me in a category that doesn't allow me a full experience. I've only had one time when someone was upset. We had a discussion with one of the leaders and I told him that telling people about myself was incongruent with who I am today. He accepted that but had felt that I should have told everyone upfront. Strange what rules the world thinks we should live by.

Even in the groups I participate in we always have an STD talk before each event. People are asked to voluntary offer information to anyone they want to engage with if they have any type of STD that is contagious. However, "we" are not "contagious" yet some people (mostly men) want this very private information provided to them. There's actually a law in Great Britain that a trans person must inform a potential sexual partner about their past history. There are actually people serving time, as of this writing, who have been tried and convicted of breaking this law.

I was with my long-term boyfriend about 4 months when he dropped the L word (told me that he loved me) and I decided that I had to tell him about my "herstory." I had not talked to him at that point about being transgendered and he had no idea. We spent a very romantic (and sexy) weekend at a blissful resort in Tucson and I told him the morning we were getting ready to leave. I told him there was something we needed to talk about. He became nervous and he told me later that his first thought was that I was a fugitive on the run or something.

He was pretty shocked, but our relationship, including the physical side, was not something he wanted to walk away from... who knew? I'm not saying this is a solution for anyone else, just that it worked for me, and with this particular relationship.

47. How did your emotional or sexual attraction affect your daily life when transitioning?

At first it didn't affect it at all. Then, about 2 ½ years into my transition, as I mentioned in an earlier question, I realized that my transition didn't feel "real." I decided I needed to explore where and how my attraction or "sexuality" was going to factor into my life. I'd always been a pretty sexual person, so I was determined that it *would* be in my life.

I almost immediately got involved with some individuals, at first in the transgendered community, and then eventually in the Tantra Community. I eventually got involved with two transgendered individuals who each eventually took their own lives. The first one died after I had known her for about a year. The second one became an amazing partner to me. I spent 6 years with him. At this point in my life I am in a committed relationship with a beautiful man who loves me unconditionally and whom I deeply love as well.

48. What did my current long-term boyfriend say when I told him?

My current and long term boyfriend, David, had a very interesting reaction to the news. I already gave a bit of a rundown but it bears telling again. After he told me after about 4 months of dating, that he loved me, it instigated me into telling him my story. I thought we were just having a good time. So I decided I had to tell him about my "past" life.

We went on a romantic getaway and had a steamy weekend and then I told him that I had something to tell him about my past. He got very nervous. He apparently thought I was going to tell him I was actually a bank robber, or wanted

90

for some crime. He never suspected the actual reason for our talk. He was pretty dumbfounded by the news. So we ended up talking for about 4-5 hours and once we talked about everything he was okay with it. It took a bit longer before he was confident about telling anyone else, but today he is very passionate both about our relationship and with me.

49. Do I like sex better as man or as a woman?

This is kind of a tricky question, because I've always enjoyed sex regardless of my gender. Early on in my life, when I wasn't dealing with the intense feelings of confusion about my gender, sex was great as a man. I would have to say, however, that I was never extremely comfortable in my skin, so now, as a woman, it feels much more natural.

One big difference is that I was much more assured of an orgasm as a man than I have been as a woman. It's been a bit of a trade off, but ultimately I would not have been able to remain a man, so it's not really a valid question to me. I find my body much more beautiful as a woman than I ever did as a man, and I like to be looked at by men and viewed as beautiful, that also contributes to my sexual satisfaction.

50. Can you have an orgasm? If yes, is it different as a male/female?

I can and I have had orgasms as a woman. I've had some difficulties since my follow-on surgery which created the hood of the clitoris and the labia, but that is another story. The orgasms I've had as a woman are significantly different than the ones I had as a man. I knew as a guy that I could achieve an orgasm if I wanted one. As a woman it seems it is not a given at all.

All of my orgasms as a woman have happened without any help from me. One happened as I was coming out of a deep sleep. I kind of panicked because I felt like I was going to explode, since my experience, as a guy, was always associated with a physical release of semen. So it was a surprise.

The other weird orgasm experience happened while I was driving. I had to pull off the road and let it pass. Both times they just sort of happened. The experience is somewhat similar but I felt the experience all over my body as a female, when, as a guy, it was pretty much a localized experience around my genitals.

CHAPTER Seven: Issues That Occur When Transitioning In The "Real" World.

51. Bathroom issues

This is one of the "stickier" issues that the transgendered community has to deal with. I actually find it strangely funny how all the transgendered issues seem to come down to this, at least on the public forum.

Frequently, when there is no other valid argument fearful people do the whole "guilt by association" thing. Throughout the 90's I hardly ever heard the term "pedophile" without the term "gay" before it. "Gay pedophile" is how certain elements of society whipped up fear and panic. They did this by simply putting whatever they happen to be afraid of before the word pedophile. I've recently noticed they are now clumping pedophile with the word transgendered, which plants fear and confusion in the "normal" population.

This also clouds the issue of transgendered individuals who just need the basic human necessity of having access to bathrooms. There tends to be a great deal of fear in the transgendered community around this issue. They are afraid of being in physical danger if they use the opposite gender bathrooms. For example, in the case of a transitioning Male to Female transgendered individual, when using the Men's room the fear is of being "clocked"; and the fear is facing embarrassment and potential legal action if using the Women's room.

It is not a problem if someone "passes" relatively well. The problem comes into play when someone does not pass very well. I have never had a problem using the bathroom of my perceived gender however that does not mean others don't struggle with this issue. I almost always talk to other women in the bathroom. It is unusual for women NOT to talk in the bathroom. I've always found smiles and conversation help other women warm up to you. The protocol for the men's restroom is quite different; there is rarely any conversation and this is especially true if one's "package" is exposed.

52. Is it difficult to find jobs when people transition?

It is very true that many Ts suffer discrimination. On the other hand, if you lose a job, make sure it IS discrimination and not a performance, relational, or personality-driven problem. Have someone call or write for a reference check on you, and see what is being said verbatim.

There are a lot of reasons why someone may get a job and not keep it long. Has he or she been doing contract work? This is common in the computer world, and companies will frequently lead employees on in believing that the contract will become permanent, then let them go when it expires and keep that built-in reason. Many companies have probationary periods specifically so that they can 'check out' a new employee before they become permanently vested in company benefits. Remember, if an employer is following the rules regarding what can and cannot be asked in an interview, plus considering that past employers usually don't give references good or bad anymore, it's very hard to get an honest performance reference on an employee. So, companies use the probationary period as a try-before-you-buy plan.

Also remember the importance of - and the weakness of - the paper trail. Paperwork must be in order - name changed with Social Security and on state ID, credit cards, etc. At the same time, never assume that an employer can't or won't find out about your past. With a Social Security number, your previous name and work history is still out there, along with any arrest records and your credit report. That old name will be there for a long time. In our day and age of terrorism and the advent of the computer it is literally impossible for the average person to remove or even restrict any old records that may be present on the Internet. Things like old work history, arrest records and credit reports with one's old name can still be accessed if someone is determined enough.

53. How did transitioning affect your job? What is the best way to transition at work?

This is one of the greatest problems facing the transgendered community today. Many have challenges revolving around having enough money to do what is necessary to transition. Money to change one's name, get hormones, keep a roof over your head, and potentially even have surgery are all vitally important issues. Not to mention purchasing a gender-change of wardrobe! I live in Arizona and there are not laws protecting the rights of an individual from being fired from his or her job for being transgendered. Sadly, this happens quite frequently.

The best option, in my opinion, is to be self-employed. This way you don't have to answer to any boss. I had my own business, and so I *am* a little biased with regards to this.

Another factor for how well one is going to transition at work is how good of an employee someone already is. It is important to be, if not *the* best, *one of the best* employees. Make yourself invaluable at what you do.

Another concern is how well you physically transition. Realistically, a company is a business and they are working to make money. Some big companies, fortune 500 companies for example, can move people around and are very dedicated to protecting a workers rights. Smaller companies do not usually have the resources to be guided by that criterion. If you are a great employee working for a smaller company, this can mediate any negative impact of you transitioning on the job.

54. What gender does your medical doctor and insurance companies consider you to be?

This is an interesting question. Medical doctors are usually very good about keeping the gender straight, although, at one point in my transition I was sitting in my doctor's office and they announced my name to go back and used my male name. I was very upset with them and the office staff was counseled about it. The insurance companies are a little different.

My medical insurance with my old company didn't really acknowledge it but I never really tested my new gender out with them. I've recently changed companies and plan to take advantage of the new insurance to get physical and other associated tests that are typically done for women, such as a mammogram. There are valid medical reasons for trans women and all women to get mammograms. Even men have been know to get breast cancer so the point isn't just to be treated like a "real woman" but to legitimately ensure that there are no issues with lumps or suspicious growths.

55. Did professionals you associate with struggle with your transition (doctors, dentist, accountants)? How do you deal with an uninformed professional?

I've kept my same dentist and he has been extremely professional. My dental hygienist, however, had to hand me off to someone else as it was beyond her ability to comprehend. That was okay; I would have been more upset if my dentist had walked away. My medical doctor was super cool and is always asking me for advice on how to deal with a wide variety of issues regarding the transgendered community. Otherwise, all the others I've dealt with, whether government, medical, or anything else tend to be above reproach.

This is always a rather complicated issue as much of how you are treated is a direct result of how you treat others, as well as how well you perceive your own fit in your world. I've met some very unhappy transgendered people who tend to "lash out" at those people in their world that don't accept them or maybe struggle with their transition. There are some transgendered folk who do not "pass" not matter how much they do to change their physical bodies.

56. Emergency services – what is the protocol (pre-op, post-op, and cross-dressers).

Unfortunately, many transgender and gender diverse people are mistreated and even neglected by members of the healthcare profession because of ignorance and phobias on the part of healthcare providers.

This has sometimes resulted in tragic situations. There is one incident of a trans woman who died because first responders realized she was trans and wouldn't provide aid. Since this unfortunate incident there is much more sensitivity to this issue. We all deserve to live and to have the same opportunity to have emergency medical care.

Medical professionals are human and can run into their own prejudices; and sometimes it can be a bit problematic for them. There are quite a few more transparent transgendered folks around now, so this has gradually improved over the years, but is still an area of concern.

As far as differences between pre-op, post-op, and cross-dressers.... NO ONE should ever be denied emergency services regardless of their presentation or how they look.

I have had a couple of experiences with this issue. Once I was stopped for speeding on my way to my SRS pre-surgery appointment. I was late and when the officer pulled me over he was quite confused by my driver's license, which had the right name but had a gender marker of "male". He was quite flustered and just told me to slow down.

A couple of years after my SRS surgery I needed a hip replacement and went to the Mayo Clinic in North Scottsdale for a consult. A new type of hip had just come out (ceramic) and I wanted that particular type. The surgeon wanted to give me the older type of hip, and informed me I was "lucky" that I had found him. He then confided in me that many Doctors that he knew wouldn't operate on "people" like me. I said, "Thanks, but no thanks." That was probably the most overt discrimination I have ever encountered. I later found another doctor who was referred to me and he couldn't have cared less about my previous history.

57. Police – What's the policy/protocol in dealing with transgendered individuals?

This depends on the jurisdiction, but in general more and more police departments are coming up with protocols on how to treat transgendered individuals. There is still a great deal of disparity on how the protocols are enforced. Generally, in my opinion, if someone identifies himself or herself as "transgendered" or a gender that is different than their legal documents say, there needs to be a "timeout" called and a supervisor should be brought in. There is just too great of a likelihood of abuse and discrimination to occur.

There are numerous documented incidents of insensitivity to a transgendered person's rights. I've only had one incident with the police, and the officer was very confused because my gender marker did not match my name or physical appearance. He called me "sir" but to his credit he just let me go with a verbal warning.

101

Admittedly, I was speeding to get to my gender-reassignment pre-surgical appointment. Fortunately, I didn't have to give him my reasons, and since he was already pretty uncomfortable I'm glad I didn't.

58. If a transgendered individual breaks the law – Boy or Girl prison?

I've been asked this question several times and the answer is pretty complex. Prisons in general are very black and white places. There are rules and regulations to handle different situations, and shades of gray tend to create confusion.
Men go to men's prisons, and women go to women's prisons. So, where do transgender people go?

Well, it depends. As far as I can tell, in most systems, those with a penis (present from birth or surgically constructed) go to men's prisons. Those with a vagina go to women's prisons. Sounds simple, right?

It is not at all simple. First, assuming that the transgender person has not been taking hormones and has not had sex reassignment surgery (sex-change operation), he or she will likely have to psychologically endure being housed in an institution for those that the person perceives as being of the opposite sex.

What if a person with male genitalia who believes himself/herself to be female has started taking female hormones before the incarceration and has fully developed breasts? Then, the person would likely end up in a men's prison. That's right, a penis and breasts, in jail with a bunch of men.

It is pretty easy to see how there are various possibilities that present challenges since transgender people do not easily fit solely into either male or female categories. Once incarcerated, regardless of the gender of their inmate peers, there are other challenges.

How can they avoid discrimination? My guess is that most security personnel in most institutions are not well versed in working with transgender inmates. People often fear what they don't understand, and there is a significant risk of these prisoners not being treated fairly. Likewise, I believe it's rather obvious how transgender inmates potentially face significant harassment, intimidation, and violence from other inmates. Many times the inmate is put in solitary confinement, which ends up being an even more punitive and severe sentence than they would normally have received.

What about hormone treatment in prisons? Should inmates who are already receiving it on the outside be prescribed these medications in prison, too? What about sex reassignment surgery? Should taxpayers bear the burden of this for long-term prisoners? Some have argued that they should.

How should one address a transgender person: as "he" or "she"? I suggest asking each person how he or she wishes to be addressed. However, I will say that every transgender person I've interacted with over the years has wanted to be addressed as the gender they felt they really were, not as the gender into which they were born. This presents an interesting dilemma in a correctional environment because referring to any inmate as "she" in a men's prison, or vice versa, elicits shocked and confused reactions from prison staff.

CHAPTER Eight: The Legal Issues of Transitioning.

59. Is it legal to change your gender?

Fortunately for US citizens, it is legal to change our gender. We can legally change our names, and there are more and more cases of doctors giving letters for transgendered individuals to even change the gender marker on their legal documents such as drivers' licenses and passports.

Legal gender marker change used to require reassignment surgery. However, over the past few years there has been some relaxing of these requirements. Due to the expensive nature of the surgery, as well as it not being covered under insurance for a large percentage of individuals, and thus surgery being so unattainable for a large percentage of transgender people, many doctors now will write letters for individuals (after an extended time on hormones) to have their gender markers changed.

Another area of discussion is legal change(s) to birth certificates. Each state deals with this in different ways. To the best of my knowledge, only Ohio does not allow modification of one's birth certificate. Some states change it and then flag the record. Some allow you to change the gender marker, but not the birth name. Some allow both, so there is quite a bit of diversity based on the different state you were born in.

The last area is in regards to getting married. As gay marriage becomes legal in more and more states this will become a moot point. However, basically it is legal to marry someone of a different gender, for example a MTF post-op can marry a man. Recently there was a case where an adult child of a man who married a post-op female contested the marriage, and a lower court dissolved the marriage, claiming that same sex marriage was illegal in their particular state. Last I heard it was heading to the Supreme Court and I have not heard the resolution yet.

One last sad and rather dark note in answer to this question is that it is NOT legal to change your gender, or even be transgendered or gay, in some countries in the world, most notable recently Russia and Uganda. You can be imprisoned for life, or even in some cases put to death, for not having a conforming gender.

60. What kind of discrimination do transgendered people face?

They face discrimination of all types. I suppose the most common is job discrimination. In many areas of the country people can be fired for any number of reasons, and so when someone is transitioning, many are either fired or just not hired when attempting to find employment. Tighter economic times result in fewer jobs and greater competition. The best thing, I think, is for people to become self-employed.

Another area of discrimination is health care. Many doctors will not accept transgendered patients, as they don't want to become known as a provider for this particular community. As I stated in an earlier question, I had a doctor I was contemplating for a hip surgery tell me that I was lucky to find someone who would operate on someone "like me."

These are probably the two most common and greatest areas of discrimination.

61. Can Transgendered Individuals be Legally Discriminated Against?

The short answer for this question regarding the majority of states in the United States is yes.

Currently, there are 21 states, which have laws specifically protecting individuals with regards to sexual orientation. There are also 17 states protecting individuals with regards to gender expression (transgendered). There are 2 states currently protecting transgendered kids. Even with states that have laws there are unfortunately many ways to circumvent the current laws.

62. Is it difficult to find healthcare providers who will work with this condition?

This is one of those answers that begins with, "It depends." I have either participated or led a support group in Phoenix for almost 14 years now. We have a rather in-depth list of providers, healthcare workers, and counselors that we know and recommend to those who ask. There are more and more counselors who are familiar with the work these days. However, this is one area of the United States. There are other areas that are still struggling to understand and be able to provide services. Sadly, some countries around the world make the whole LGBT dilemma illegal and prosecute those in the community and those who try and reach out to them.

CHAPTER Nine: The Nuts and Bolts of Transitioning – Hormones, Surgeries, And Mental Health.

63. Is There a Recommended Order To Transition?

There is a recommended order and it's based on the Harry Benjamin Standards. Many people go in all kinds of different directions based on their life circumstances, and this also varies slightly if the transgendered individual is a female to male, however, the following order may not be the exact recommended sequence per the official Benjamin Standards but is my first hand recommendations based on my transition.

The first step for anyone considering transitioning is consulting a therapist, preferably one with experience with the transgendered community. Being transgendered is what's sometimes called a "self diagnosed" condition. Sometimes therapists diagnose it as well. It is imperative to deal with any other possible psychological issues not associated with being transgendered first. Many therapists in North America require individuals to take the MMPI (Minnesota Multi Personality Inventory).

After a certain amount of time with a licensed therapist's guidance and a medical Doctor's supervision, hormones are prescribed as the next step. A letter from a therapist to the Doctor is all that required to being taking the medication. Most start with partial doses and after a short period of time are then upgraded to full doses of hormones. Hormones are, in my opinion, one of the litmus test of being transgendered. Therapists say that if someone goes on the hormones of their perceived gender and have a bad reaction, then it (being transgendered) may not be what the problem is.

The next step, if the person transitioning is financially able, is to begin hair removal. This can be the most time consuming step so should be started as soon as possible. It can also be done concurrently with all the other steps.

The "Real Life Test," is the next required step. This test involves living in your perceived gender for at least one year, and should be carefully planned. I've met numerous individuals that I have known have had to "change back" because this step wasn't carefully planned. This is probably the most important step of all. This step has to be successful in order to actually be able to make the transition a reality. It's very important in this phase to seek out help through group counseling and support groups that can help you with this phase. Seeking out help and support during the test is very normal and healthy and does not imply weakness. A wide variety of things need to happen during the test. In my case: I saw a counselor every week, I changed my name, I began electrolysis, I began to plan how to finance any surgeries than I thought I would need. Bringing family and friends on board through education and loving understanding is essential. This process is the actual real life experience of living in your perceived gender.

At some point during "The Real Life Test," depending on the effects of the hormones, personal preferences, and of course financial constraints, a decision regarding surgery is the next step. For MTF, some people do facial feminization, some do breast augmentation, and most do reassignment surgery. Not everyone gets surgery. 75% of Male to Females do not actually get surgery for a wide variety of reasons; some just want to live their lives in their perceived gender and do not need surgery to do that. For the FTM, during this phase hormones have a significant role. Facial and body hair begin to grow, voices deepen, and there are usually tremendous physical changes that take place from the effects of the hormones. There are also some decisions to be made with regards to surgery. The percentage of FTM's that actually have surgery is much lower than the MTF's. It is estimated to be 3-5% that have any type of surgery at all. Mastectomies are typically the most common surgery that they have.

After surgery there are a myriad of other psychological issues, such as depression, confusion about how to live the rest of their lives, their roles in their families, dealing with the physicality of their new bodies that have likely arisen, and sexual attractions that were not dealt with in the process of the physical transition. Making massive change is always difficult, however if the goal is to change one's gender then the above sequence is a typical path for many transgendered individuals.

64. How does one go about picking a new name?

This is an interesting question. I am always interested in how someone picks his or her new name. I have met some MTF transsexuals who have hated being a man and want nothing more than to get as far away from their given name as is humanly possible. These group of individuals usually pick what I consider to be very feminine names such as, Tiffany, Stephanie, Jennifer and so on. They also tend to have issues with men in general, whether that stems from dislike or fear.

Others pick names similar to their male names or even incorporate their old names into their new names. Most psychologists agree that the more one can integrate their past lives into their present lives the better it is from a psychological point of view. I've also met some transgendered individuals who have chosen names that their parents told them they were going to call them if they had been born the other gender. The more your can get your family to participate in your journey in ways like this, the less likelihood you will have of them rejecting you.

So my male name was Dean. When I first began to transition I tried to make is as similar to my male name as I could. The first name I came up with was Dena. My rational was I the same person just with some "things" rearranged. Unfortunately, I didn't like the way it was pronounced, Deena. So I began to look for another name and I like the name Anna but I knew someone who had already picked that name. It was my mother finally who helped me decide on the new name of DeAnna. She even suggested that I capitalize the "A" so that people would pronounce in correctly. I also thought that it would be a good analogy of, "I am the same person, with something added." It is not uncommon when someone is either contemplating a transition, or is early in their transition, for them to change their name. Sometimes the name just doesn't fit.

Names are quite important, and most people transitioning put a great deal of thought into their new name and it is important to honor that. One of my uncles summed this up quite nicely one day. He told me, "Well you'll always be Deano to me." He thought he was being supportive but I told him that it was insulting. One of the reasons we transition is to get to the right gender for ourselves. However, if the world ignores everything we have gone through, we can still feel like a prisoner in our own bodies when anyone refuses to acknowledge this amazing transformation. My uncle did start calling me by the correct name after that. He didn't understand this, but he did it; and I truly believe people want to help but just don't quite know how.

Once the new name is picked it is time to legally change your name. This varies from State to State and basically entails filling out paperwork and then going before a Judge. If an individual is married or divorced with minor children they have to sometimes get written permission from their spouse/ex-spouse to ensure that they are not trying to evade ex/spousal responsibilities such as debts or paying child support. Check your state and local guidelines to see the procedure in your state and country.

65. How long does it take to transition?

Everyone tends to transition at his or her own pace. The Dr. Harry Benjamin Standards say that at a minimum a person has to be on hormones and living in the role of their perceived gender for a minimum of 1 year before having surgery. These standards apply in the United States but do not necessarily apply in other places around the world. Even here in the states I've seen people transition in as little as 6 months. I've met others who have been "transitioning" for over 20 years.

Once the decision is made to change, there is typically quite a sense of urgency to complete everything fast. I like to say it's like climbing on a fast moving train. The problem with this is that the families and support system for each individual sometimes need more time in order to keep up. I spent about 4 years transitioning and a great deal of that was working with my family to try and keep them on board.

Taking this time allowed my family to participate as well. My younger sister took me to get my ears pierced for the first time. I brought my entire family in for a group counseling session once. There were many emotional moments, and because I took the time it was an experience that brought my family together. All too often this can be something that causes families to explode or even reject the individual completely. This is an altogether too common occurrence with transgendered individual's families.

Bottom line: we all continue to grow and change as human beings and the growth hopefully always continues.

66. When you made the decision, did you weigh the pros and cons and then decide?

In my experience, changing genders was unlike any previous decision I had ever made. This was a decision based on the heart, not the head. The only logical decision I made was whether I would live or die. While I'm not trying to be overdramatic, I believe once you decide to "not be yourself" you begin a slow death.

This is especially true in my case. I believe I would have "died inside" if I hadn't chosen to go down this road. That being said, I honestly didn't see any way to stay physically alive if I would have had to keep my old form, as a man in my case. I've heard of gay people who stay in the closet who end up dying young because they can't live the right life. I've come to realize that when you suppress anything you tend to make it stronger. It also "slops" out or manifests in a myriad of different physical problems, ranging from heart disease to cancer.

67. Is that your real hair?

Yes. Many transgendered people have real problems with hair loss. There are operations to move up the hairline and get hair plugs, which can become very expensive. Going on hormones actually can help the situation, and I've heard of some people who have had some regrowth but in general once it's gone it's gone. I was lucky with the gene pool. I don't have any problems with hair loss and both of my sons have great heads of hair. Some genetic women also have problems with hair loss so it's not just a one-gender problem.

68. How did you get rid of the body hair?

This is one of biggest challenges for many MTF's. I spent 3-4 hours a day, 3 days a week, for almost 3 years straight going to one of my best friends for electrolysis. It is painful and tedious. About halfway through I almost had a nervous

117

breakdown but was able to make it. I spent probably close to $30,000 with electrolysis, and that was just my face. I also got approximately $6000 of laser hair removal for my body. The reason there is such a disparity in cost is that facial hair is much more resilient than body hair. Think of just the texture of a beard versus the hair on the body. Body hair is generally much softer and less coarse. For me, one of the biggest confidence boosters as a female was when I didn't have to shave anymore.

The biggest problem of hair removal for my generation is that we have some grey hair and they tend to be the hardest to get rid of. My friend Maria would always say I wasn't the hardest one she had ever seen, but then after I was done I overheard her say that, in fact, I *was* the hardest she had ever done. I'm just glad she didn't tell me that when I was in the middle of it.

69. What are the difficulties with wardrobe/shoes/etc...

This really depends on the body types of the individuals who are wearing them. Sizes are different. Women and men use a different system completely. In general, men have broader shoulders, wider waist sizes, and larger feet and hands. Amazingly, hormones can change some of these things, but overall the key is to try things on. There are some on-line retailers that actually cater to these communities. Some stores like Payless do carry some larger shoe sizes. Again, it's important to just try things on.

70. What are some of the effects of the hormones, both immediate and long term?

In my case, the hormones had a tremendous effect on my body. It all depends on one's genes. Some people get great effects from the hormones, and some experience little to no effect from the hormones. This is really a complicated subject so I must say these are simply my experiences with hormones. I am no expert on the subject other than how it relates to me. That being said, making the decision to go on hormones was a big deal to me.

Hormones are kind of the litmus test as to whether you are transgendered or not. As a MTF transition, if you have a bad reaction to the hormone estrogen, then you are likely not transgendered. I had a friend who went on estrogen and it put him on an emotional roller coaster and after a short time he decided that this was not the thing for him. Hormones really are the first concrete step on the road to transitioning from male to female or vice versa.

I have heard amazing stories about hormones. I've met some sisters who say that the day they went on hormones everything changed. The sky was bluer, the flowers were brighter, and they had a powerful awakening. My experience was a little different. The first morning I started on hormones, they gave me my initial doses of the various meds and I received an injection of estradiol. This occurred at around 10am.

I did not experience any of the things that they said I would experience, however, at about 4:30 pm, I was laying on my bed watching a rerun of a TV series called the "The Pretender." At the end of the show I just began to cry and cry, which was bewildering to me because it wasn't really a sad show. I had flashbacks to one of my wives crying before going to bed and I kept asking her, "what's wrong?" She proceeded to tearfully tell me, "I don't know." When I was a guy, if I would have cried every day I would have thought I was having a nervous breakdown. Now, if I *don't* cry every day I feel like I'm having a nervous breakdown.

71. Are physical changes from hormone treatments reversible?

For trans men (FTM), there can be significant physical changes if taking testosterone in Hormone Replacement Therapy (HRT).

- HRT does in most cases result in increased body hair growth and in some cause head hair loss as well.
- Skin can become thicker and voice can drop.
- Features can become significantly masculinized.

For trans women (MTF), HRT often includes antiandrogens in addition to estrogens and progestogens. HRT causes potential infertility, among other changes HRT does NOT usually cause facial hair growth to be impeded or the voice to change.

- Potential infertility if taken long term.

Partially reversible changes

- The growth of breasts with concomitant enlargement of the nipples (may need reconstructive surgery to reverse the effect).

- Redistribution of body fat as well as some thinning of skin.
- Infertility, eventually leading to chemically induced aspermatogenesis. The reversibility of this effect depends on the length of time and effects of androgen suppressing substances. Androgen suppressing drugs are not a substitute for other birth control methods.

Reversible changes

- Decreased libido.
- Redistribution of body fat (in most cases).
- Reduced muscle development.
- Various skin changes
- Significantly reduced and lightened body hair.
- Change in body odor and sweat production.
- Less prominence of veins.
- Ocular changes.
- Reduced gonadal size.

The psychological changes are harder to define, because HRT is usually the first physical action that takes place when transitioning and the act itself of beginning HRT has a significant psychological effect, which is difficult to distinguish from hormonally induced changes.

72. Do transgendered people go through another adolescence period like teens go through?

Absolutely! Just like young men and women in adolescence, it's about finding your niche of who you want to be and what styles suit you. There is some aspect of "social rebelling" involved, and this may show up as miniskirts in MTF's and lots of leather in FTM's. In general this does not take as long as in younger people, since most transgendered have already experimented to some degree with these things, but I have known some who get stuck in this period and never really move out of it.

73. Are transgendered individuals required to seek counseling?

If a transgendered individual is seeking to have reassignment surgery, they are required to be seen by a licensed counselor. To actually transition they are required to have two letters of recommendation from counselors with masters-level degrees.

This is the requirement, but from a pragmatic point of view there is so much involved with transitioning that everyone needs someone who can help them deal with all the issues that may come up. I've known transgendered individuals that have "gone it alone" and they never truly deal with all the aspects of transitioning.

The more support an individual has, the smoother and more successful their transition is. Many individuals are still adhering to the male stereotype of not needing anyone. This is a lie and will ultimately not serve the individual transitioning. Support groups can also be extremely helpful. Avoid spending time with negative groups or individuals who spend a great deal of time dealing with all the "pain" of transitioning.

74. Is there a special type of surgeon who performs reassignment surgery?

There is no formal title for the doctors that do these types of surgery. The ones that do it exclusively tend to be what I call hybrid surgeons who specialize in plastic surgery and urology. This is due to the nature of the surgery as there is some "rearranging" of the patients "plumbing," so to speak. Ten years ago there were a limited number of surgeons who did the work, now there appear to be more and more doing it. I went to a surgeon in the Phoenix area who specialized in this surgery because I wanted someone with lots of experience. These types of surgeons generally cost somewhat more than less specialized surgeons, because they are simply better at what they do.

75. Is surgery for transgendered individuals covered by insurance?

This is a controversial topic. In general, most insurance companies do not yet cover it. Some larger companies are beginning to cover the surgery, most notably Intel Corporation. I do believe it will eventually be, covered by insurance. I think a good comparison is gastro bypass surgery. Most insurance companies now cover gastric bypasses, as it is considered to be a "once in a lifetime" surgery. The SRS (Sexual Reassignment Surgery) is also a once in a lifetime operation, but it will likely take time for the general population, and more importantly the insurance companies, to accept and ultimately pay for the operation.

The surgery is a big obstacle for most transgendered individuals. There is quite a bit of stress and anxiety about this life change, and without the final surgery many people are condemned to live a life of being stuck between genders. They may be able to live transparently as transgendered, but many would ultimately rather be their perceived gender. Partially transitioning allows individuals to live and work as the correct gender but can be a huge impediment to getting into relationships. Many transgendered individuals choose not to get into relationships for this reason.

As of this writing it appears that Medicare will begin to cover the surgery in the coming months. This will be a tremendous help for those who have not been able to afford the surgery in the past.

76. How long is the surgery, and the recovery time after the surgery?

My surgery was 11 ½ hours long. Depending on what you're having done it's usually less. I did not want to have to go back into surgery in a relatively short period of time, so I had it done all at the same time. I had rhinoplasty (a nose job), breast augmentation, and, of course, the SRS (sexual reassignment surgery). Each one lasted about 3 ½ hours.

I spent approximately 9 days recovering in the hospital. One of the things that are required is to dilate at least 5 times a day for about 10-20 minutes. The new vagina will collapse on itself if it isn't "exercised" every few hours. This decreases as time goes by but its still recommended daily unless you have regular sexual activity (which I do). The recommended time is 4-6 weeks of recovery. I was actually back to work in about 2 weeks, so again it just depends on a person's age and how relatively healthy they are.

77. How did it feel to have "it" cut off?

This is usually the point where I talk about the surgery. I like to say it's a very "green" operation. Most everything in recycled. Nothing is, per se, cut off. I usually describe it in very simple terms. The skin of the penis is harvested and becomes the lining of the vagina. The clitoris is formed from the super sensitive nerve cluster at the head of the penis. The only parts that are "throw away" are some erectile tissue and the testes. Everything else is recycled. It's more complicated than that but those are the essential facts.

78. Are silicone injections for breast augmentation suitable for transitioning trans women?

Silicone injections are once again legal in the United States. Silicone breast augmentation was banned for a period of time due to an autoimmune issue, which has since been found to be unsubstantiated.

I have seen good results with both types of breast augmentation material (saline and silicone). When I had my surgery, silicone was not available, so I have saline and have been very happy with them. If something were to happen (leakage or rupture) I personally preferred to have that be saline, which could be absorbed into the body. Silicone is not something the body manufactures naturally so I had concerns regarding how my body would deal with this substance. There was quite a bit of bad press about silicone at the time I was considering my options and that weighed heavily on my decision. However, it was also not available so it was a moot point. I've heard that silicone has a more natural feel to it than the saline implants. I have never physically compared them.

79. How did your view of your physical body change?

As a woman I am generally much more conscious of physical attributes than I was as a man. I have always had a space between my front teeth; this never bothered me until I started transitioning. I had my dentist fix it. I also changed all the fillings in my teeth to white as I became much more aware of my smile and that I wanted it to look good. As I began my transition I also lost a significant amount of weight. I wanted to wear the "cute" clothes and not the baggy stuff that larger women have to wear. I immediately began to grow my hair longer and got really into facial products.

80. Is there a voice surgery to feminize your voice?

Transgender voice changing is a complicated process that requires three factors to achieve success. A strong understanding of the process will give you the greatest chances of achieving a voice that sounds natural and is perceived as female by others. The first step is understanding the differences between "pitch" versus "voice" versus "speech."

Pitch is simply the frequency at which the vocal cords vibrate, and determines the frequency of a sound produced. Pitch is essentially ALL that the voice box (larynx) does. The pitch at which we speak is called the fundamental frequency, and the array of pitches our larynx can produce is called our range. An untrained male voice usually has a little over an octave (equivalent to 12 notes on a piano scale) of range.

Surgery to raise the pitch of the voice, known as feminization laryngoplasty, is relatively straightforward in most patients, in experienced hands. Having the final voice perceived as being female, rather than just a higher pitched male voice, goes well beyond pitch-raising surgery.

Voice is what results as we mold the sounds we produce. Voice is determined by the size and shape of our throats, mouth, nose, and sinuses, giving it resonance, just like the size and shape of the piano which houses the strings changes its sound. The "voice" or sound of an upright piano would sound different than that of a concert grand piano even if the same note were being played. It is important to understand that the resonators of your voice, the shape of the throat, mouth, and sinuses, CANNOT be changed in feminization laryngoplasty. Even gender reassignment surgery and/or facial cosmetic surgery CANNOT change these resonators. Assessing these areas pre-operatively is vital to predicting how the voice might sound (and be perceived) afterwards.

Next, voice is shaped into words and sentences. This is speech. A genetic female uses a different part of the brain to produce speech than a genetic male, and has a certain singsong quality called prosody. This is what the brain of someone listening to you will subconsciously process, and perceive the voice as being female versus a high-pitched male voice.

Visual cues are also very important, but for the purposes of this discussion, visual cues are assumed absent, such as with telephone conversations. Prosody CANNOT be changed with hormones or surgery. It must be learned, the way an actor would acquire the skills to take on another's personality. It requires a speech therapist, who is experienced in transgendered voice changes and can teach prosody. In most, it also requires practice to perfect the new speech habit and have it sound natural and effortless.

Perfecting prosody is 50% of the final results. This is why a genetic female with a very low speaking voice is still perceived as female, even when their pitch is in the male range of fundamental frequency (such as many female television reporters).

I chose not to have this surgery as I felt it was not as important as other things. I spent quite a bit of time and effort working on my speech. There are many techniques to affect the change; you just have to seek them out. The easiest is finding a DVD or CD about voice feminization, getting a small voice recorder, and experimenting with your voice. Singers sometimes have a better result because they tend to have more experience training and manipulating their voices.

81. How did you change your voice?

I did not have voice surgery. There are some procedures available, but they are pretty ineffective as of the last time I looked into it, especially in the male to female transition. Speaking is a very complex thing, and the biggest "tell" for us is not necessarily the pitch of our voices, but rather the resonance of our voices. The best solution is still some voice training with a professional voice coach, or even some really good CDs about how to speak with a more feminine voice.

My voice seems to be fine in person; however, I still have some struggles on the phone. Without the physical cues people make snap decisions based on intonations in our voices. It's kind of funny how the slightest differences in our voices, especially on the phone, have people making decisions about our gender. Normally I answer the phone and give my name right up front and that usually allows people to get it right.

82. Did you have to learn new habits and mannerisms?

I think initially I kind of learned some basics, like sitting with my legs crossed, which I've been told by girlfriends, is body language for "I don't want sex." Overall I don't really think I changed a great number of things. Most women cover their mouths when they, cough, sneeze, eat, and burp. I guess you can say I just started to be a little more polite. I say excuse me and I'm sorry more often.   I think you have to do what comes naturally to you. I have some friends that make very strange over-exaggerated hand gestures. One new, and unexpected, habit is to always check and make sure my dress isn't stuck in my underwear after going to the bathroom.

CHAPTER Ten: After Transitioning – The Good, The Bad, And The Ugly.

83. When you saw your breasts for the first time did you just stare at them for hours?

There is a funny story about this question, which of course, a guy asked. The only request I had for my doctor about this before surgery was "Not too big." Speaking in reference to my new breast size. When I saw them for the first time they looked huge, and my first comment was, "holy shit, I'm gonna kill someone!" I was still feeling pretty dopey from the drugs, but when my doctor came in on his rounds he saw my look and immediately commented, "well, the girls said, 'she's pretty broad shouldered, she can use a little more'" (saline in my implants). So I said to him, "who are these girls, and where do they live? 'Cause I'm gonna kill 'em!" After I healed I did start working out and shaping them, and ultimately they turned out pretty nice, so no one had to die .

84. Did you ever contemplate suicide... before, during, or post-surgery?

I, personally, did not ever contemplate suicide. My parents did have some concerns about me, as

I did deal with quite a bit of anxiety when I began to contemplate the overwhelming challenges of transition. I have, however, been touched by it repeatedly. I have had two intimate partners commit suicide. Anytime anyone commits suicide it has devastating results, but when it is a partner or spouse it can leave tremendous suffering behind. I was with my last partner for over 6 years when he committed suicide.

I have met other transgendered individuals who make it all the way to surgery and then after surgery either attempt or commit suicide. I've always struggled with this more than anything. Transitioning seems to be such a consuming experience for some, that when the journey is over, i.e. post-surgery, it's like people don't have a reason to live anymore. That seems really strange, but I have seen it happen several times.

An article in the Los Angeles Times in January of 2014 showed a whopping 41% of people who are transgender or gender-nonconforming have attempted suicide sometime in their lives. This is nearly nine times the national average, according to a sweeping survey conducted in 2011.

Researchers are digging deeper into that number and analyzing the results of the National Transgender Discrimination Survey in order to examine what puts transgender people at such "exceptionally high" risk. Researchers from the

American Foundation for Suicide Prevention and the Williams Institute at UCLA School of Law found that the risk of attempting suicide was especially severe for transgender or gender nonconforming people who had suffered discrimination or violence, such as being physically or sexually assaulted at work or school.

85. Did you worry about going out in public?

Yes, I did have tremendous fear about going out in public. When you make such a major physical change, it's probably human nature to think, "everyone is watching." I still remember the first time I "successfully" went out in public. It was in the spring of 2000, and I went to a meeting in a strip mall, at a wig store, and I was terrified.

Prior to that, I had an "unsuccessful" outing around Christmas of 1988. I was in the military at the time, and had purchased my first wig. I was walking downtown and a group of young men "clocked" me. Clocking is the term that we use to describe when someone identifies us as being transgendered. This group of young men began to yell at me, but they were driving past and were unable to stop because they were on a one-way street. They went further up to turn around and I took that time to reverse my route and get lost in a parking lot. They were unable to keep up with me. That incident set my transition back probably about a decade, and made me think it was not possible for me to change my gender.

86. Did you have any "ah ha" moments?

I've had numerous "ah ha" or epiphany moments. I suppose the first one was the moment I realized that becoming a woman was actually possible. That moment in time that I made a decision to believe that transitioning was even possible was a huge revelation. I have since come to learn that this how we accomplish anything in life, making a decision to believe that whatever "it" is, is, in fact, possible.

Another big moment was realizing that, in fact; no one was actually "watching" me. Nobody really cared what I was doing, as long it didn't impact his or her reality. I suppose the biggest epiphany I had was that, at one point, fairly early on, I was struggling with men looking at me at the mall. I brought this up with the women in the band I was playing in. They proclaimed that it was just what men did; they looked at women and they were usually pretty rude about it. I did kind of a headshake and said, "You mean they're just checking me out?" My girlfriends said something about all men being pigs and so on.

"Well," I said, "I'm going to check them out right back!" I lost most of my fear of men on that day, and it was very liberating and lightening.

Another breakthrough I had was the realization that when people would come at me about their fears *for* me, they were really just mirroring their own fears. I learned a *huge* lesson somewhere in this mess that when something in me upsets or angers someone that it really isn't about me but rather their own internal issues that I am bringing to light. As human beings we all have ideas or realities that we believe to be true. The list is exhaustive; the issues come up when something or someone comes along that challenges these "truths."

It is said that whenever something new comes into the human consciousness the first thing that happens is people ignore it. The next thing that happens is they laugh at it. The next thing is they respond (sometimes violently). The final thing that happens is that things become self-evident. This is happening with gay marriage, it happened with equal rights, it happened even with giving women control of their body (birth control and abortion rights), and to some extent it is now happening with transgendered individuals.

My new attraction to men was also a rather significant moment. My counselor had told me that attraction was a little more fluid than most people believed. He also told me that our attraction usually was tied to our dreams and, more specifically, whom we dreamed about. My dreams had begun to involve men and it was not too surprising that I eventually was drawn to men more and more. I did not really lose my attraction to women, and ultimately I came to the realization that I was now, for all intents and purposes, bisexual.

87. How have your hobbies changed?

I like to think that none of my hobbies have changed, although I suppose some have. I think I did some things because of an innate need to feel masculine. I let go of those rather quickly, however, many of the things I liked before transition I still like to do. I enjoy getting out in nature, I love camping and hiking, I love to target shoot, and drive fast. I've always liked to cook and bake. I like to clean and do laundry. These were things that were forbidden for me to do as a child, so I guess I developed an appreciation for them simply because I was not allowed to do them as a child.

I do not like to sew or knit, and probably never will. We had a trans woman in our group for a while who thought that those hobbies were necessary to being a woman. There are so many preconceived notions about what it means to be a woman, or a man, today. None of them matter other than the ones that each individual feels is in their best interest.

88. Did your transition solve the problems that you thought you had?

Transitioning did, in fact, solve at least the most pressing problem that I had. I couldn't focus anymore and just spent so much time and energy trying to decide what to do about my gender issue. Once the gender issue was resolved I was able to focus again and go back to living my life, although so many things changed that I kind of had to figure out what living my life actually meant now.

What was important to me before transitioning; things like work, family, and church, began to evolve into other things. I became more focused on learning new skills and finding out what I authentically felt called to do.

Now, roughly ten years after transitioning, I have a new career, new interests, new ideas about spirituality, new love in my life, and am still learning more about myself. I am more curious than ever and want to try things that I simply want to do, rather than doing what I feel like I *should* do. I am now doing things that I would have never imagined, like studying Tantra, practicing meditation, writing books, and making music.

89. Do you ever have doubts and wish you hadn't changed?

Since my prior life seemed like such an untenable situation for me, it does little good to wonder what if. Sometimes I think I would have had better relationships with my sons. There is just no way to know. I've heard of other, even prominent, transgendered individuals who have advised others to not do it (transition). They advise others to take medication but do not transition. I think everyone has to walk his or her own path and see where it goes. One person's solution is not necessarily the right way for anyone else.

I've talked to several counselors about this topic and there are several reasons for some to de-transition. It is usually tied to other problems the individual has. I've found that there are surprisingly more reasons to transition than just the most obvious one of feeling conflicted in their gender/body. I've met people that literally hate themselves and are willing to do radical things to get away from who they are. These people usually back away from surgery, as that is kind of a huge litmus test about what the problem actually is. There have been a few incidents of people who have regretted the decision to have surgery, however, due to the relatively strict requirements to have counseling and therapy pre-surgery, this is relatively rare.

90. How have your physical surroundings changed?

My physical surroundings have changed significantly. I like being surrounded by beauty and so my home these days is full of my tastes in pictures and decorations. I really did not think about my surroundings that much before changing my gender. Much of what I decorated with was just "stuff" left over from my kids, military days, and just minutia that had no bearing on who I really was. I now have a very thought out scheme to my home. The wall next to my bed is full of butterfly pictures and memorabilia. There are romantic and dreamy pictures as well. It's funny because I was rather oblivious of how it affected my daily mood before I became aware of how important my surroundings are.

91. How does hearing the wrong/right pronouns affect me (During transition and post op)?

Hearing the right pronouns, especially in the early stages of transition, is extremely powerful. Hearing the wrong one can actually be very difficult at this stage of transition. I tried not to be too affected by it, but there were some significant incidents that happened that made me feel very frustrated and in despair. I had a very good support system in place, but there were still some rather heated moments when someone would refuse to call me by the right pronoun. My daughter Katie was a huge advocate for using the right pronoun, especially within my family, and I will be forever grateful to her. Post-operative I have never been called by the wrong pronoun except occasionally on the phone, and then I just gently correct them.

92. Did surgery change the way you perceived how people perceived you as a person, subconsciously?

Yes. Once I had the surgery I felt complete and congruent. This resulted in a huge shift in my psyche because now everything lined up; my physical body, my brain, and my spirit were now all one. I can't speak for anyone else but I would have felt trapped if I had stayed in my old form. This is why we have so many addiction issues, depression issues, and suicide issues.

The hurdle of trying to cope with incongruence between our hearts, minds, and bodies results in a tremendous amount of fear; Fear of the world, of being discovered, of relationships, and so on. I believe that we energetically reflect to the world what we feel inside. When someone is conflicted it is often perceived (even if only subconsciously) by whomever they are interacting with.

93. Do you now feel more confident?

Yes. I was confident before surgery, but having the surgery gave me a huge boost. After surgery I felt like I could walk through the world without anyone being able to question me about who, or more importantly what, I was. I was mistaken about the last part as I'm still occasionally asked the "what" question. I usually tell people I'm either a Democrat or an alien. I still find it a little mind-boggling that people don't feel a little weird about asking me my gender. Fortunately, it rarely happens anymore.

94. Is there anything you miss about not being born a woman?

Mostly the answer is no, however, there are some things that I do wish I could have experienced. One would have been childbirth. I would have at least liked to have the option as to whether or not to actually birth children. Feeling new life inside of myself, creating a new human being. The whole experience is something I would have liked to be able to do.

Overall, I think it's an advantage to have lived a male life first, but sometimes I have trouble connecting with other women on topics ranging from abuse to just feeling insecure. Unfortunately, I have been sexually assaulted, and so I've had more experience in common with the typical woman than I had previously thought. One of my first experiences working in my last business as a real estate appraiser involved my client following my around and not trusting my ability to do the job. I've also experienced not being taken seriously at an auto repair garage.

95. Do you miss the masculine supremacy? Now a 2nd class citizen.

I was actually asked this question at a support group meeting recently. It's interesting because we do live in a patriarchy; I was just surprised that the question was even asked. The answer to this question is "no," because in the context of being who we are and/or who we are trying to become, it becomes irrelevant.

If I am a woman then any advantage to being a man was just a temporary condition anyway. NOTHING is more important than being authentic and true to whom we are. This is also similar to being a Christian. I enjoyed being a Christian and feeling like I was part of something bigger than myself. However, at some point I outgrew my fellow's Christian beliefs, and even though I felt a little scared at leaving the "flock," I had to authentically follow my heart and my growing beliefs, which eventually led me in a new direction.

96. Is the world different as a woman? Do you view the world differently as a woman? Do you feel yourself being subjected or objectified as woman?

The world is a very different place for women. I would have never believed that we live in two different worlds, but now I can say irrevocably that it is true. So many things changed for me in a practical sense as well as a spiritual sense.

I had a business as a real estate appraiser when I transitioned. One of the things I did was drive around and take pictures of homes. As a man, I was often looked on suspiciously when I was doing that. I would wave and smile but it didn't seem to make a difference. After transitioning, most people waved at me first and even stopped me and wanted to know what I was doing, not in a hostile way, but as if they wanted to connect with me.

I do view the world differently, and I am a much more peaceful person these days. I am horrified when the country goes to war. Things I wouldn't have given a second thought to before sadden me now. If I had cried every day 10 years ago I would have thought I was having a nervous breakdown. Nowadays if I don't cry every day, then I would feel like there is something wrong. My tears seem to be my barometer and I pay very close attention to it.

To some extent I feel both objectified and subjected. At this point in my life, it actually validates my journey, but it can be annoying. My first time out appraising as a women I was followed around and watched very closely. The client assumed I didn't know what I was doing. I do not get taken as seriously as I would have been as a guy. I've been told to "calm down", and not to get so emotional. Women, however, have many tools at their disposal that men don't have. In my opinion and life experience, beauty and subtle sexuality are very powerful tools that most women rarely learn how to use effectively. There is a stigma against women that use their sexual power in this way; however, some women in the pursuit of "equality" with men tend to overlook the effectiveness or even the power of using their beauty and subtle sexuality to achieve their goals.

97. How have your worldviews changed?

I had been a military officer and businessperson for a long time, so I would have described myself as a solidly right wing conservative Republican. As I transitioned, I developed so much more compassion for all of humanity. I literally went from being a staunch conservative to a very "bleeding heart liberal". My counselor and I were talking about it one day, and he made a statement that, while there wasn't much difference between the parties these days, he felt that Democrats were more interested in "justice and fairness" than the Republicans. I realized at that point how many of my prior political views I had developed solely because of my role as a man. After making that realization, I almost immediately changed my party affiliation and began voting my conscience rather than my gender or past persona. It was a very liberating experience.

98. How have my views on men/women in general changed?

I have so much more compassion now for both men and women. Looking back on my, life I would say that my attitude toward men was that I mildly resented them and wasn't sure why. I've done some regression hypnosis and have had some personal revelations. I can't speak for anyone else, but what I now believe to be true was that in my past lives (yup, past lives), I've always been female and have dealt with numerous episodes of rape and losing children to male aggressors.

I was a Christian for many years and so neither of the concepts of "past lives" nor K
karma/dharma was on my radar screen, up until sometime within the past 4 years. I believe I came around this time as a man to resolve the latent anger/rage within me. I actually began to do this while I was in the Army by gradually starting to see the inner child in most men. I learned to enjoy their energy and appreciate what they bring to the table.

I've also always enjoyed being around women, and felt I was one of them. As a child, during the holidays I remember always joining the women in the kitchen and listening to them talk. My mom would try and shoo me away to go hang with the guys, but I found the "other boys" boring and uninteresting. I loved being with a group of women. In high school I also always had many more friends who were girls than guys. I can only remember having one good friend who was male.

99. How are you treated differently now?

At some point, and I'm not really sure where or when, I stopped comparing my different experiences and just began to enjoy my life. I am accepted and treated like a woman no matter where I go. I always get stopped at the airport because I have an artificial hip, so I have to get "special" treatment there.

It's my belief that, in many ways, women are treated better than men overall. I find it is a kinder, gentler world for women. I've had so many good experiences of men holding doors for me, talking to me and just being kinder. I also enjoy that women just so easily bring me into their confidence; and since I now have so many "female" experiences in common, I rarely am at a loss or unable to connect to anyone, male or female.

100. Is life easier/harder as a woman?

This is another question I get asked that is somewhat hard to answer. It was very difficult to be a man because I never "felt" like one. That fact alone made being a man "hard." I was always struggling with my "inner demon" or woman. Being a woman is easier than I thought it would be because it just is so natural for me to be one. Having such a huge internal difference, whether you are woman or a man, results in you always being conflicted, or incongruent, within your own skin.

Like many boys, I spent a great deal of my time between the ages of 11-14 trying to figure out what it meant to be a man. I was told (by parents and other role models) that I had to put away my feelings at that point and somehow figure out how to make the best of being a man. Since being a man didn't feel authentic to me, I read hundreds of Westerns that talked and gave examples of what "real" men were supposed to be like. Things like honoring and respecting women, being honest in my everyday life. They were a bit old fashioned but were nevertheless what I incorporated in my understanding what it meant to "be a man."

The cultural differences are too numerous to point out, but they pale in the face of not being whom you perceive you are supposed to be. For me, the bottom line is: when you are happy in your own skin, everything in life is easier.

101. Any correlation between changing your gender and bad/good things happening to you?

Life is life. I've had many good and bad things happen to me. I am a Life Coach now and I've come to realize that really nothing is implicitly good or bad. Everything that happens to us has a purpose and is showing up in our lives because we need to grow, in some way, as a human being. This has been an amazing journey for me and I have learned so much about myself, and human nature in general, that I now see the need to categorize between good and bad as irrelevant.

102. Do different generations deal with this dilemma differently?

My experience leads me believe that the answer is, of course, yes. My generation (baby boomers) had very little if any information about what this was. I spent quite a bit of time trying to comprehend it and even trying to decide if I was gay or not. I always kept coming back to the fact that I was attracted to girls, even in my younger years.

Because we were unable to get better information about it, we came up with all kinds of ideas. My first thought was that I felt this way because I associated with women. So my first solution I ever came up with was to go into the military so I wouldn't have to be around so many women. We now know that such is not the case; this idea falls into the category of the "garbage in, garbage out" problem solving technique. False assumptions lead to false conclusions.

There was also quite a bit of fear in how my generation dealt with it. I used to laughingly think to myself that I would have to shoot the first person I told because my life would be destroyed afterwards. The good thing about my generation was that most of us went on and had pretty conventional lives. We got married, went to college, found careers. We did what everyone else did and in the process, as most people do, we became problem solvers to some extent. This was very helpful to us because when it became necessary to transition, many of us just went at it like any other problem in our lives.

I've had quite a few dealings with the next generation. Generation X (or whatever they're calling it these days) had just enough information to keep them from really going out and doing what the baby boomers did (ignore it and live a "normal" life). They had their own ways of dealing with the issue. Most I have met did not get into relationships; they tended not to go to college, most seemed to just sort of be waiting for the inevitable to happen. The problem was that many of them didn't really learn how to problem solve.

When they finally felt like they needed to transition they were unable to because they didn't have the resources or the will that the baby boomers tended to have. They also tended to not have very good family support, although that is always the joker in the deck no matter what the generation.

The next generations have unique issues as well. There is a younger generation of what I call "gender benders" who just kind of express any way they feel like. There are also issues involving the younger generations that we didn't have to deal with, like the possibilities of getting on hormones and stopping puberty. This generation as well as the "X" generation lacks a very important ingredient, and that tends to be "confidence". There seems to always be this need to try and "make it" as the gender we are born as. I'm not sure if this is innate or if it is cultural but seems to transcend generation boundaries. It may be that, the older you are, the more personal power you have to deal with the societal ramifications of transitioning your gender.

In conclusion, no generation has it easy. They all have their good points and bad points, strengths and flaws. It's always a challenge and we just simply have different ways to deal with it.

103. What have I learned, overall, from going through this transition?

The main lesson I have learned as I've transitioned is that we all have some purpose on the planet. I've personally learned how to love regardless of the circumstances. I've learned that people don't necessarily want to be afraid, and if we come part way they'll come the rest of the way. I've learned that virtually nothing is impossible if you believe it's possible. I've learned to never take life for granted, and to be grateful every day for the amazing experience we are having, even when it's hard to be grateful.

CHAPTER Eleven: How Do I Support Transgendered Kids – Good Things to Know.

104. What should parents do if they suspect their child is transgendered?

This is a complicated question. For those of us who are transgendered, most (but not all) know as early as our first conscious memories that there was "something" wrong. However, due to long held societal and religious beliefs about gender, immense pressures to conform cause almost an immediate need to hide it from one's family. It should easy to understand that conflict may and usually does occur between us and our other family members. If understanding and acceptance is not given relatively quickly most of us experience considerable stress. We may be uncomfortable, embarrassed, nervous or afraid. We may be desperate to find and grasp "solid" answers. Our discomfort impacts the entire family. So the best thing to do is find a good therapist and confirm what is going on with the child and help them guide you. Most importantly remember to listen to the voice of the child. I always felt so validated when TG children started showing up on the national forum.

The answer to this question is a little disturbing and not what you think.

On Feb. 20, 2012, the American Academy of Pediatrics released the disturbing, but unsurprising, results of a long-term study investigating abuse rates among transgender children. The investigation followed some 17,000 people who demonstrated "gender nonconformity" before age 11, measuring their mental health and markers for abuse in early adulthood. The findings of the study were alarming and indicate a frightening and hidden epidemic of abuse.

Their parents had abused a full 39 percent of transgender men and 30 percent of transgender women. Most of the abuse victims demonstrated signs of post-traumatic stress disorder, a very serious condition marked by severe anxiety and suicidal ideation.

As a transgendered woman, an LGBT activist, and as a result of having many friends who are transgendered, I feel personally troubled, not only by the degree of abuse among transgender kids, but also by the fact that it has gone relatively unnoticed.

Recently, the parents of transgender children have been in the media spotlight, and attempts to discredit, attack and insult these parents are common. The mother of Bobby Montoya, the 7-year-old transgender girl who joined Girl Scouts last year, has been a subject of threats and organized boycotts. Seattle's Cheryl Kilodavis, author of "My Princess Boy," has been continuously attacked by the right-wing media. A lesbian couple in Australia was the subject of international debate when they allowed their transgender daughter, Tammy Lobel to transition at age 11.

These parents have become famous for "abusing" their kids by embracing their children's identities. When a parent actively supports her child's "deviant" gender identity, she is considered to be corrupt, sick, "politically incorrect," and guilty of brainwashing her child. Yet the tens of thousands of parents who have physically, sexually, and psychologically abused their transgender children go unreported by the news.

There is something severely wrong with our society when it is headline news for a mother to allow her male-bodied child to wear a dress, and especially when she is considered abusive for doing so. It becomes societally endorsed abuse when a headline like "Mother Spanks Son for

Wearing Make-Up" is unremarkable and uncontroversial. We live in a world where abuse of transgender children is substantially more common than support, and this is problematic and dangerous.

The epidemic of abuse toward transgender youth must end. Of the many adults I know who are transgender or gender-deviant, I know very few who have not experienced child abuse, and even fewer who do not suffer from long-term mental health problems because of this abuse. For the health of future generations, we need to ensure that this problem ends now. The parents of transgender youth owe their children nothing short of full support, unconditional love, and a stable family life.

106. Why did it take so long for my child to tell me about their transgender identity?

The simple answer to that is fear of rejection. I have heard one horror story after another of families that have rejected their transgendered child, to the point of concluding that this is probably far more likely to be the norm than acceptance. As a country, we tend to be very freaked out about sexuality in any way, shape, or form. Most children, even as adults, do not want to risk losing their families. It takes tremendous courage and self-confidence to be able to "come out" to friends and family.

I used to, in jest (sort of), say, "I would have to shoot the first person I told because otherwise my world and life would be over." We talk about the crab bucket affect, where we all work very hard at keeping the people close to us from doing anything that changes our concept of them. This is also a contributing factor to why we have such a high suicide rate in the transgendered community. It can sometimes be a very lonely road to go down.

107. As a parent is there anything I could have done to prevent this from occurring?

Parents ask this question often. The simple answer to this question is, no. There was some speculation, at least with my generation, about a drug that was prescribed in the 50's that caused more transsexual babies to be born. DES or Diethylstilbestrol was, and still is, theorized as a possible reason for babies being born with this condition. However, the drug was banned in the 60's and there are still many transgendered babies being born around the world.

I believe everyone has a purpose for being on the planet and we all have different paths to follow. Being transgendered is one of those paths, and our job, like everyone else, is to try and discover the way. It does little good to try and second guess what we could have or should have done to prevent some type of birth anomaly. It serves us so much more to see how the world needs the gifts that we bring to the planet.

108. Should transgendered kids and/or their families seek counseling?

Therapists differ dramatically in their approach to these children, with some taking the relatively new approach of supporting kids who want to live openly as members of the opposite sex. Others encourage kids to discard their more pronounced behaviors, explore new interests and embrace their birth gender.

Many therapists take the middle ground, for example; accepting a very determined boy's desire to wear dresses and saying it's fine for him to do so at home, but strongly encouraging him to refrain from that behavior in school, where he might encounter unpleasant responses.

"I think the general trend has been to take more of a stance of tolerance toward the behavior instead of the old type of stance where they would yell at (these boys), criticize them, punish them for any sort of girlish behavior and send them off to military schools," says Gregory Lehne, an assistant professor of medical psychology at the Johns Hopkins University School of Medicine. "That didn't work particularly well." The reality is that a family's reaction varies considerably beginning with the parents; ranging from acceptance of child's difficulties and some realization that everyone is different and has his or her own developmental pathway, to less accepting. The bottom line is that these children are very conflicted and they are often traumatized and bullied by other children at school.

109. When do you think kids/people are old enough to change their gender status?

I know that you would like a quick and easy answer to this question. But, as with many issues in life, the answer may be quite complicated or reveal itself over time. For most children, the answer is very simple. When given two choices -- boy or girl-- most kids feel strongly that they are one or the other. However, some children cannot so easily make this choice, and when given a wider set of options, will provide a wider set of responses.

When your 18 month old girl's first words are "me boy" or your two year old son insists he is a girl, and these responses don't waver over the next few years, you can be pretty sure that you have a transgender child. This does not mean the second a child demonstrates behavior that is inconsistent with their biological sex you should assume they .are gender nonconforming. But if you can look over time and see that your child has persistently and consistently made that assertion, it is probably not just a phase.

So the answer is: whenever the time is right. There are some very young transgendered kids that are quite happily transitioning while young, some as early as they can talk. There are some that are being put on puberty delaying meds until they reach the age of 18. The best advice is to try and honor what the child is telling you and let them be your guide. In many situations adults think they know what is best for their child and most times they are right. This isn't one of those times. Transgendered kids (like all kids) want love and acceptance from their parents. They will try very hard to be something they are not to try and keep their parents' love.

I did not know what my condition was as a small child, but I just knew very early (age 3-4) that my parents would not understand my dilemma and, even worse, I couldn't tell them about it. I learned in a very painful way (embarrassment) that my family would not understand. I went on to live a quite productive life, but ultimately I could not continue living as my present gender when I felt so torn on the inside with who I was on the outside.

110. How can I be supportive of a transgendered friend, family member, or partner?

Simply be there for the individual. In so many cases the first thing that happens to someone who comes out about being transgendered is that their entire support system walks away from them. I remember how difficult it was at the church I was attending and how just one person after another would come to me crying or desperately trying to keep me from transitioning. I heard over and over again we are so "afraid" for you. Of course, we know that it's not the individual that we are afraid of but rather our own internalized fear about our own sexuality or identity.

111. What is the best way to address a transgendered person?

I have literally never met a transgendered individual that wanted to be addressed differently than how they felt or were presenting in public. On that note this is an easy question to answer. Address a transgendered person based on how they are presenting. So what do you do with someone giving off "mixed" signals (such as androgynous apparel)? Engage them in conversation and simply ask them how they want to be addressed. It's usually taken well if you're curious, and as long as the question is sincere.

112. Is it true that some people who have transitioned do not consider themselves "transgendered"?

This is true. There is a large and growing community of "post-op" transgendered women who consider the term "transgendered" as irrelevant. Logically, if all the different aspects of someone are lined up, heart, mind, body, and spirit then the term just isn't accurate anymore. I remember at one point I was paying more and more for medical insurance and when I called them and asked them what the deal was they said I had Gender Dysphoria. I told them that in fact I had been "cured" and was just a plain old woman now. After I sent in the proof of my surgeries they then dropped my premium by 2/3.

I like to say that being transgendered is part of my "herstory," but is not who I am today. This is turning out to be a bit of a controversial subject these days. Interestingly, Great Britain has passed a law requiring transgendered individuals to divulge their previous history to any possible sexual partners. I consider this a huge invasion of privacy and am also once again risking transgendered individual's lives because of irrational fear from the general populace. There have already been some individuals convicted under this new law.

I've personally encountered dangerous situations; such as when a man I was with became very belligerent and said that he felt "tricked." Luckily he calmed down and we had a very long conversation about it. I explained that I didn't tell him my past gender, because now I am just being authentically who I am. Everything matches up in me. We finally came to an amicable agreement. For me, divulging this aspect of who I once was compromises the integrity of who I am now.

113. How do transgendered people go about changing their gender?

I can only speak for myself, but you change your gender like you do anything else in life. For me, changing my gender is something that percolated throughout my lifetime, and it became very evident, especially during the last 5 years before I chose to transition, that I couldn't avoid living as my authentic self any longer.

So, the first things I recommend you do are research it and develop a plan. I began seeing a licensed counselor (this is required) who had experience with this particular issue. After seeing him for a few months, and much soul searching, I went to see a doctor who also had experience with the transgendered community.

On the recommendation of my counselor the doctor prescribed hormones (estrogen and a few variations). Hormones are the litmus test and one will find out quite quickly if they begin to create problems. If someone is transgendered, getting on the right hormones will give them peace of mind; if it's wrong for them, then it will create lots of anxiety and just plain angst. I hear many interesting stories from other people when they go on hormones, like the flowers were prettier, the sky was bluer, the air smelled fresher, and so on.

My only unique experience with the hormones early on was that after seeing the doctor in the morning and receiving the different medications, I laid down on my bed, as was my habit after working most of the day, and after watching a show on television I began to cry and cry. It was very disconcerting and confusing as it wasn't even a really sad show. It called to mind a time when I had found my wife crying one night before bed and asked her what was wrong, and she said, "I don't know." Anyway, that was my "welcome to hormones" incident.

After I was on hormones and had gone to weekly counseling to prepare me (and my family) for about 6 months, I made the decision to legally change my name. This was another big decision point for me as this began what is called The Real Life Test*.

*This is simply the requirement for an individual to live as their target gender for a minimum of 1 year. This is, of course, just hypothetically a "test" because it is not a pass or fail situation, and there are many different resolutions to this process. I just always thought this was a funny name for it, because what if you "flunk" the test?

I remember my counselor asked, after one particularly frustrating week, "Do you want to go back to being a guy?" I immediately said "NO!" That ship had sailed some time ago. This question helped me to stay focused on who I wanted to be, and not be swayed by whatever issues I was complaining about at the time.

Around this timeframe I also started electrolysis. I believe this is the one experience that really separates someone who is confused about their gender with someone who is willing to do whatever it takes to change their gender. I spent a little over 3 years going 3 times a week at about 3 hours a session getting the hair off my face and body. I came close to a nervous breakdown toward the end of this process, as it was painful, expensive, and I was losing hope that I would ever be done with electrolysis. I became best friends with my electrolysis provider, Maria Denacoli, who was there for me at this critical moment. She changed my appointments to early in the morning because my pain tolerance was much higher earlier in the day. It was the only way I was able to finish.

I spent about 2 ½ years transitioning. The requirement, based on the Benjamin Standards, is 1 year in one's perceived gender. I went as slowly as I could, mainly to enable my family to remain on board and continue to support me.

I've met several transitioning individuals who went too fast and their family ended up having to walk away. My daughter at one point told me that if she could have seen where we are today at the beginning of my transition she wouldn't have been able to come with me. Because I went slowly, the old question, "how do you eat an elephant" is very relevant.

I had some experiences with sexuality towards the end of my transition. I personally needed to know where my attraction was heading, At that moment in time I had begun to feel that my transition wasn't real and needed to see what life after transition was going to look like. Many transgendered individuals do not need to know this before transitioning.

The next thing was to come up with the money for surgery to complete my transition. My wife and I had decided get divorced, and so over the previous years we had settled up and I was able to refinance my home to pull some money out, enough to go to the surgeon I wanted as well. So just short of 4 years after changing my name I was able to have the surgery. I was able to finish up with the electrolysis about 2 months after that.

I was back to work full time about 3-4 weeks later. This is a thumbnail sketch of how someone transitions. There are other issues, like attraction and relationships, that were not part of my narrative, but these are the essentials of physically changing ones gender. In addition, there are some legal aspects to consider.

I have never regretted changing my gender. I have met some individuals who actually regret going through the transition. I have heard of others who have changed back to make a partner happy. I don't stand in judgment of those individuals as I have always known that people change their gender for a variety of reasons, not all being because they feel conflicted. Some change just because they do not like who they are.

I continue to help lead a transgendered support group and speak at universities occasionally about my journey from male to female. I've participated in a number of projects regarding videoing some aspects of my transition.

I'm a bit unusual in that I have been in relationships most of my life (including my life as a woman). Many of the transgendered people I have encountered do not end up having long-term relationships. I believe that as human being we all seek connection and relationship with others. Many transition and then decide to live a solitary life assuming that no one would be able to deal with his or her story. I have found that to be completely inaccurate. We all have stories and we are no different in that respect than anyone else.

The most amazing thing I have done since transitioning was to quit my job and become a life coach. I have done so many amazing and "impossible" things that I literally don't believe in the word "impossible" anymore.

Four years ago I lost my long-term transgendered boyfriend, Michael, who committed suicide January 4, 2010. He was a combat medic in the US Army and had served in Iraq. He went into the service for many reasons but had slowly become more and more desperate to get out and transition. He was struggling with PTSD from the Iraq tour and had tried committing suicide a little more than a year previously by jumping off a bridge in Italy, where he had been assigned after serving in Iraq. After a year spent in grieving and trying to find reasons to get out of bed every morning I decided to make an important life change and became a life coach.

I decided to do an intensive 15-day immersion type of course in Sedona, AZ. On the first day of the training, which was phenomenal by the way, I met a woman (whom I refer to as the Purple Girl) who I was immediately magnetically attracted to. It was very strange in that I was physically attracted and simultaneously repelled. She was at the training for about 5 days and I was completely confused by her and what I felt about her. I found out while she was there that she was a Tantra practioner.

I had never heard of the word "Tantra" before and became very intrigued with it. Before I knew what it was I "felt" the word. I found that it is actually many things but one of the meanings is about the balancing of Male and Female energy. Who knew? Another was the practice of "sacred sexuality". Both of these subjects have always fascinated me. The Ying Yang symbol represents this energetic balance within all humans of male/female energy.

After some deliberation, I realized I was incredibly drawn to the practice of Tantra; so much so that I went to Hawaii and studied with Sasha and Janet Lessin to become a tantra practitioner. Tantra has been a life-changing journey on the sexual side of being transgendered. Interestingly, transgendered people actually embody this whole male and female energetic struggle that everyone has, but few every really delve into. Most transgendered people sadly, never are able to reestablish themselves as sexual beings.

I've met so many amazing people on the Tantra path, not the least being my wonderful new partner David. He is another life coach and

Tantra enthusiast and we've been together about 2 1/2 years now. Another is my close friend, Tracy Elise, of the Phoenix Goddess Temple.

I've been able to keep my immediate family with me on the journey. We all worked very hard to stay together. My experience is that families that try and disconnect at the beginning of the journey rarely are able to reconnect later on. My daughter not too long ago informed me that if you could have seen where we would have to go ultimately, she probably wouldn't have been able to come with me. It's the whole, "How do you eat an elephant? One bite at a time," scenario. I have 3 kids all in their 30's now, all have their own lives. I also have 11 grandchildren that I love very much. I am in their lives as much as they allow and as much as I want.

I sometimes look back at my life as a guy and really wonder at how I was able to accomplish so much while struggling with my intensely conflicted internal nature. It seems surreal at times. I rarely tell anyone I meet in passing about my previous life as a man. Most don't want to know and I really feel no need to share, but will eventually if a relationship is destined to become long term. I'm one of the transgendered individuals who does not recognize being "trans" anymore.

Spiritually, I was a born again believer for many years and I helped lead a Christian Worship Team for over 10 years as a transgendered woman. After discovering life coaching and a host of other metaphysical disciplines I can only describe my most recent experience, as transcending Christianity. Some might consider me a mystic as I see the commonality between all religions.

I met my current life partner at the Phoenix Goddess Temple while attending a Naked Life Coaching session with Nadine Sabulsky, and have for the last few years been involved in the Science of Mind community. Christianity is my foundational spirituality but once I opened up to the vastness of all that is spiritual it's next to impossible to go back to one narrow aspect of it.

Another interesting aspect of my interests lies in feminism. I have become a huge advocate for women's rights. I kind of thought I would be an advocate for men but am stunned by all the subtle persecution of women even in America, not to mention around the world. I suppose it's the whole "walk a mile in someone else's shoes" thing.

Overall, I still have the daily struggles everyone else has but I am now living the life I believe I was intended to live.

Thank you for reading my book. It is my hope and intention that I have been able to help you in your quest for answers to some of the questions surrounding what it means to be transgendered.

I am available for public speaking on a variety of topics ranging from sexuality and gender, to how to overcome the impossible things in your life.

You can reach me on my Facebook page at: https://www.facebook.com/awakeningstreams

Or my website:
awakeningstreamslifecoaching.com

www.ingramcontent.com/pod-product-compliance
Lightning Source LLC
Chambersburg PA
CBHW071353280526
45787CB00001B/302